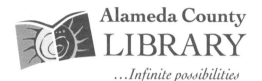

Cockeyed*

Cockeyed

A MEMOIR

Ryan Knighton

PublicAffairs
New York

Book design by Jane Raese
Text set in Bulmer

Library of Congress Cataloging-in-Publication Data
Knighton, Ryan.
Cockeyed : a memoir / Ryan Knighton.
p. cm.
ISBN-13: 978-1-58648-329-6
ISBN-10: 1-58648-329-3
1. Knighton, Ryan—Health. 2. Retinitis pigmentosa—Patients—Biography.
3. Blind—Biography. I. Title.
RE661.R45K64   2006
362.197'7350092—dc22
[B]
2005058697

FIRST EDITION

10 9 8 7 6 5 4 3 2 1

For my gal

My purpose is to tell of bodies which have been transformed into shapes of a different kind . . .
—**Ovid,** *Metamorphoses*

Contents

Prelude

Every Sunday, when I was a kid, my family drove to the out-
skirts of Langley, British Columbia, my hometown. My
grandparents worked a hobby farm there, just this side of the
U.S. border. My uncle and his girlfriend would show up, too,
even my great grandparents who arrived at pushcart speed in
their immaculate Parisienne. Our Sunday dinners at the farm
were the best of plain British fare—Yorkshire pudding,
whipped potatoes and gravy, roast beef, the works, and I
loved every mouthful. Every taste of those days.

The farm was everything my two brothers, my sister, and I
could have wanted—pellet guns, cow shit, electric fences,
horses, and a dying Toyota pickup we abused at high speeds
around the back acreage. Driving always devolved into spinning doughnuts in the tall grass while my siblings clung to the
roof and tailgate.

When I was in my early teens, my Uncle Brad was somewhat of a hero to me. He had long hair and a 1980s anthem-
rock moustache. He stood six-foot-six, drove an orange
souped-up Chevy Nova, and stockpiled porn mags under his
bed like cords of firewood. What more could a boy admire?
I didn't notice that he'd bummed around until he was thirty,
only that he gave me an acoustic guitar when I was twelve.

My uncle also played bass in a band, a band called—wait for it—Bender. My Uncle Brad, Nova-driving Brad, doing rock duty with Bender. Here's a man who refused to age. That resistance is what I grew to admire most. He did not go gentle into a good benefits package or practical footwear.

Because I admired him so much, it stung even more the night he mocked a sprouting oddity in my face. I was at a cruel threshold in puberty. I wanted to be seen more as a buddy than a kid, an equal of sorts, and therefore I wanted, more than anything, to be cool in Brad's eyes. I needed to be—I don't know—Bender-worthy.

The entire family sat around the dining table, digging in. I had a mouthful of perversely bitter brussel sprouts when my uncle made a face at me, a stupid Popeye look with a cartoony tone to match. It's hard to be seen as a potential roadie when your hero teases you like the five-year-old he still takes you for.

"Aaargh," he said, all piratey and probably stoned. "You be mocking me with that face of yours? Wipe that look off your face, or I'll do it with me forked hand."

He pulled his left hand up his long shirt sleeve. Only his fork poked out. Stuck on the end, a thin piece of ham flopped about as he gestured. I couldn't help thinking of the meat as a piece of face he'd wiped the look from. The idea made me want to ralph more than the sprouts. I puzzled at his pirate impression, then looked around the table to see if anybody knew what the hell he was on about. Nobody seemed to get it.

"What?" Brad said. "Look at his face. Ryan's got a squint

or something, in his left eye. See? He's kind of cockeyed."

Everybody swung their gazes my way and stared. My mother was the first to agree, making the *oh yeaaaah* noise of concerned recognition. Someone mused that the brussel sprouts caused my new look, and someone else said I got winking half right. In the culture of my family, jokes and sarcasm express one of two things: affection or worry.

I excused myself from the table and tried not to run to the bathroom, but ran anyway. It was true, what Uncle Brad had said. My left eye squinted back at me from the mirror, its top eyelid dropped lower than the right one, relaxed and half drawn, sleepy and inert. I forced it open, pulling my face back into balance, but when I reposed to my normal feeling of expression, the left lid dropped down again. I must have worked at righting it for a good fifteen minutes before my mother knocked on the bathroom door.

She asked to have a look. Nothing hurt, I explained, and nothing seemed out of focus, either. I couldn't even feel myself squinting. Ma said she'd make an appointment with the eye doctor and reassured me it was probably nothing. Ma's side of the family have gimpy, weak eyes. I already wore coke-bottle lenses. They probably needed upgrading to binoculars, that was all.

Since nothing else could be said or done, we returned to Sunday dinner. Its usual rumpus carried on, but I felt a little freaked. My uncle winked at me to make amends for his pirate joke. Then my little brother, Rory, whined about how Ryan gets everything and how, if I had a squint, he should be allowed to have one, too.

Ma took me to the eye doctor the following week. My new prescription didn't curb the cockeyed look, though, and the doctor couldn't detect any further trouble. Not to worry, he said. Maybe I had a muscle spasm. That would pass. The matter was set aside and soon forgotten. To balance my face, I adopted a sleepier, half-lidded look. The camouflage worked. Nobody seemed to mind the change. But I did, and my squint persisted, always there, as if trying to focus through a problem I couldn't see. Not yet.

Heavy Metal Diagnosis

VLADIMIR: *"I'm asking you if it came on you all of a sudden?"*
POZZO: *"I woke up one fine day as blind as Fortune."*
—Samuel Beckett, *Waiting for Godot*

In 1987, at the age of fourteen, I landed my first full-time summer job. It was so cherry. All my friends endured the usual suburban grunt labour and franchise humiliations, but not me. Five graveyard shifts a week Jason pumped gas, most of it into the monster trucks of beer-sodden cowboys. Among other paranoias, his clientele accused Jason of shooting them amorous looks. Never wipe a windshield too cheerfully. Other friends of mine, countless McFriends, as we called them, manned the front lines of military-style fast-food stations. The brand names had arrived, and they pressured the shrinking farmlands of Langley. Naked parking lots and mal-nourished strip malls began to pock the landscape. Soon they became a more frequent sight than the old, decaying dairy barns or lush cranberry bogs. But what did we care? We were fourteen and broke. Everything new was ours. Each franchise was a summer job, and each was a place to go, to find your friends on Friday night, if you weren't working. Eat and kill time. We were a new fast-food order.

My summer job introduced a fresh paradigm. I took off into what seemed the most elite niche of rare and exotic careers known to me or my friends, a real job, an occupation of mystery, promise, and serious responsibility. I was a teenage shipper-receiver.

At $6.50 an hour, I was also two bucks ahead of everyone I knew. As if riches weren't enough, the Help Wanted ad I spied in the *Langley Times* promised that driving the forklift would be a primary duty around the warehouse. Here I was, only fourteen, already driving, required to drive, and getting paid for it. They called this work? Fortune had smiled upon me, I thought, a rich and toothy grin. My father spent most of his working day driving, too, pricing commercial fence installations around Vancouver and its suburbs. At the time, I liked to imagine us both poised at the beginning of a transformative summer, one in which we would discover a new bond in work and exhaustion, not just father and son anymore, but fraternal working stiffs with weird tans. You know, the kind drivers get from hanging one arm out the window. That was going to be my summer. That and weekends of shaking myself stupid in bumper cars. I'd earn money driving a forklift, then spend it crashing at the amusement park.

My employer was Great West Pool and Spa, a manufacturer and installer of outdoor pools and hot tubs. They did everything from sewing vinyl pool linings to engineering spas for maximum massage and kinky effect. A plain, blue phrase hung on the wall in the shipping department, each letter stylized in an ocean wave motif—We Work For Your Leisure. Nobody but me was quite that naïve. Could Great West Pool have sold water and bubbles as accessories, they would have. A customized licence plate hung on the owner's frugal mini-van. It described him as a "SRVIVR." The phrase meant to capture his survivalist, free-enterprise spirit but only conjured in me images of a man who had successfully driven his Dodge through a nuclear blast.

My cheer over the forklift was premature. Because I was new, for my first few weeks on the job I didn't drive anything. Instead, I rode the forks—or, more accurately, clung to them—while Pat drove, often with me hoisted near the warehouse ceiling. Up there I scanned the hundreds of neatly shelved boxes of folded pool linings for the right invoice number. When I found it, I dragged and pushed the two-hundred-pound cardboard box onto the forks, grunting and cursing, sometimes outright pleading, as if the liners could be motivated. All of this took place about eighteen feet in the air, in a precarious balance. In action, I was like a carnival sideshow, a man forced to combine walking the tightrope with wrestling the fat lady. But it didn't bother me, not as much as it should have. What bothered me was Pat, particularly when he locked the brakes and gutted himself laughing. I had to clutch the forks for my life.

Chewing him out didn't help. Once I did my best to muster some command in my barely pubescent voice. Imagine Scooter from *The Muppet Show,* his four-eyed geek fury, seething, all pinch-voiced and nasal, imagine him really laying in and giving you shit—then you may have something close to the androgynous power I managed.

"Pa-at!" I whined, "Pa-at! Fucking cut it out! I'm gonna fall! Do it again and I'll—do it again and I'll tell Greg."

"Pa-at," he mimicked, "cut it out, Pa-at, I'm gonna fall."

My father had warned me about this sort of thing, indirectly, through years of suppertime stories about his own warehouse goofing. Life on the shop floor is a culture of whimsical cruelty. You have to play along or die. Often they seemed to be the same choice. I remember eating dinner when I was seven or eight and my father recounting over a spoonful of beans and wieners how he and the other grunts had spent the previous night's graveyard shift at war in the parts yard. For kicks they'd jimmied the safety switches off the pneumatic nail guns and had themselves a shootout, each guy positioned behind an oil drum or bails of heavy gauge wire. Later they calmed it down a bit and just shot their lunches. The morning shift arrived the next day to find bologna and peanut butter sandwiches crucified to the lunchroom door. Warehouse work can be serious horseplay, I learned. Now I was on the forks, my loyalty in question, a hint of hazing in it, to be sure, and I intended to make my old man proud.

"Here, I have a good idea," Pat continued, with what could only be a bad idea for me. "Let me help you down so you can go tell Greg your big sob story."

He ground the gears into reverse, punched the propane, jerked us into motion, and locked the brakes again. The forks swung violently back, rearing the machine like an aggravated horse. The force flung me against the greasy steel face of the lift. I imitated moss, and clung.

Looking back, I know Pat's play was helpful. Though I hate to admit it, he schooled me swiftly and absolutely in the laws of this new culture. After that, I thought twice about snitching, and my place in the order of things clarified. That is, I was on my own, and there was no order of things. Well, none aside from having the upper hand or being subjected to somebody else's. You were either on the forks or behind the wheel, and that structured your day in a rhythm of ambush and survival. Part of my job was to take it on the chin, my chin usually pressed to the cold oily steel twenty feet above Pat's shit-eating grin. Besides, how could I rat to Greg after mopping my own brain off the floor?

The forks rocked back and forth and eventually settled. Pat kept on trucking with laughter. Pat in his sleeveless Slack Alice t-shirt and high purple nylon shorts, hockey-hair Pat, Pat who made me sweep the parts aisle while he smoked behind the assorted diving boards. Pat who, one week later, backed the forklift into the SRVIVR van.

After the accident, he was suspended from all forklift duties, except riding on the forks. That was fine with me. Somebody had to drive. I was next in line and a natural choice, I thought, not necessarily out of poetic justice but because I had, for some reason, also made misreading the big, black felt invoice numbers a bit of a habit and an irritation for Greg.

I liked my boss, Greg. He was in his late twenties and had worked at Great West for five or six years. A farm kid, he had an almost oppressive work ethic. Somehow he also convinced us this ethic set a just and reasonable expectation. Not too many other bosses could do that. I had to admire him and suffer his example. Work was just something you did, no complaints, no wasting time pissing and moaning about it. If I whimpered about the heat in the warehouse, he'd say, "I'm so sorry. Would you prefer to work tomorrow when the weather is more suitable?"

From anybody else that would have seemed blunt, but you were reminded, by Greg's manner and tone and by his example, always in the warehouse himself, sometimes simply sweeping and tidying when things were slow, that work by any other name was duty, and duty is hard to dodge without sacrificing respect. Greg bull-worked days at Great West Pool, then helped his father nights and weekends with the care and handling of their family's two race horses. Labour, in short, was the key to much of his character, and I had to respect him for it.

Greg's sense of humour, like Pat's, was physical, but it lacked the cruelty I'd come to expect when I was on the clock. Greg went for theatrics, often loading a semitrailer in Monty Python character or breaking into weird horsy sounds and galloping boxes between warehouse and truck. I never knew what to do with that kind of acting out. It was embarrassing, nerdy, but it was a relief. Maybe his humour was a farm kid thing, too, because it made sense as a way of working. All that hop-to-it left little room for play, so his sense of play had to be as physical. It had to integrate itself into the task at hand. You couldn't stop to tell a joke; you couldn't just drop what you're doing to shoot your lunch. No time for that. But a strange whinny and a gallop actually got the boxes into the trailer and seemed to entertain Greg and the rest of us at the same time.

Greg was also observant. I learned that by becoming a subject of his study. It began one day when he stopped calling me Knighton, opting for the more editorial "Bumbleton." That was the day Pat's forklift keys landed in my hands. It wasn't without some debate, though. Greg was reluctant to let me drive, so I finessed him, giving it my teenage rhetorical all.

"So, like, do I get to drive now, or what?"

"Whoa there, cowboy. I don't know if that's such a good idea," Greg said, stroking his thin moustache.

Pat, Greg, and I sat around the dirty lunchroom table, pictures of buxom Miss June on the calendar behind me. We were well into July. Pat leaned back in his chair CEO-style, his grubby high-tops on the table, his legs crossed, and his eyes pinned to the calendar. A smug smile pulled at the corners of his mouth. The expression clearly attached itself to the thought that either I wouldn't get the plum job of driving, or he might get it back at my expense. Evidently either option satisfied.

"C'mon, Greg, you said I could drive soon, and you need someone to drive now."

"I dunno. I dunno if you're a good gamble. You're a bit of a bumbler, Bumbleton. You have to admit you miss a lot of stuff."

Pat's smile broke loose and he let out a guffaw. "Bum-ble-ton."

Greg knocked Pat's legs off the table. "You're a pig. You know that, don't you? A pig."

"Better than a Bumbleton," Pat jeered, "I'd be a pig before a Bum-bleton."

Time would measure Pat to be twenty years old, but part of him remained back in those developmental years when the word "bum" is a thrill.

I didn't know how to defend myself. "What do you mean I miss stuff? I work hard, don't I?"

"Yeah, you do," he said, "but although Pat here is an accident, a walking, talking error, you are accident-prone, and that's not a good thing to put behind the forks."

Pat nodded with sage and serious agreement.

"C'mon, you must have noticed it," Greg continued. "Sometimes you trip over stuff right in front of you, like that box of scraps this morning, the one that was blocking the door to the sales office. Or, like the other day, when I pointed to that case of PH chemicals and said, 'Knighton, grab that for me,' and you're like, 'Grab what?' And I pointed again, and I'm like, 'Grab the case right there. It's right there, sitting in the middle of the aisle,' and you're like, 'Where?' It makes me crazy. Then there's the matter of taking down the wrong liners. I don't know if you need your glasses checked or what, but, for chrissake, you get them wrong more often than Pat does, and—"

Greg paused, perhaps sensing he'd crossed a line, gone from presenting his reasons to ranting. I was burning red, embarrassed and confused, which hadn't been his intention, so Greg tried to repair the damage in a way we could all appreciate. He inflicted damage elsewhere.

"I mean, you read them wrong more than Pat, and you and I both know Pat's illiterate, so I want you to stop making him look good."

Pat shot up from his chair and scowled. "Fuck you, Greg, fuck you and your love for Bumbleton." He stormed out of the lunchroom and humped back down to the shipping area. Within minutes our boom box belted out Pat's favorite hurtin' ballad, Led Zeppelin's "Black Dog."

I knew two things at that moment. The first thing I knew was I didn't want to work as a shipper-receiver for the rest of my life. Warehouse work was hard, crappy; the pay was lousy; and the Pats outnumbered the Gregs. The other thing I knew, and didn't want to admit, was Greg's insight. He had hit the target when he called me a klutz. I knew deep down he was right. How could I account for it? I hadn't always been inept, not at home, not at school. I commented when Judy in sales cut her hair; I caught footballs; I had a good eye. So, I did the next best thing to explaining my flubs. I tried to worm my way out of them.

"The liners," I began, "it's just that it's so dark up there. It's hard to see the numbers, you know? It's black felt in the shadows, that's all. And the box I tripped over, I was carrying a bin of filters and I couldn't see around it and then, well—but I pay attention, Greg, and I work hard—"

Greg's lunch still sat untouched on the table between us. He took a sandwich out of the brown bag and began to unwrap it. "I never said you don't work hard, Ryan. You do." His tone shifted. He became quieter, concerned even. "If hard work was an issue, Pat would go before you. But I just don't know if I can trust you behind the wheel when you are, well, so clumsy. Sorry to say it, but I don't know what else to call it. We need someone to drive, though, a lot of orders to load in the summer peak weeks, so I've either got to trust you behind the wheel or hire somebody else, and that'll cut into your hours and Pat's hours, unfortunately."

He took a bite of his sandwich and chewed, not looking at me. I didn't know what else to say, so I waited. Greg finished his lunch while I stared at Miss January and Miss February on the wall behind him. Great West Pool was not living up to its promise. My job was making me into a strange and ham-fisted version of myself, one suspended between the beginning and end of the school year. I felt like I was dangling from the tips of a forklift. My first summertime blues.

Greg crumpled his lunch bag and shot it basketball-style into the waste bin, then broke into a Monty Python voice.

"Oh, hello, sir. I came here for an argument. Do you have one, an argument? I would like an argument, please."

"No," I muttered. "I don't. No argument from the feeb."

"Well, sir, Sir Feeb, let's just say I like you, so we'll just skip all the argument for now and see how you do for the next few days. You drive, just do your best, and most of all—and I mean it—pay fucking attention fucking all the fucking time, sir."

As I said, I liked Greg.

"And stay away from boss-man's van," he added.

I did. I gave it my best for the next few days, and I paid all the fucking attention I fucking could fucking pay. As promised, I did it all a safe distance from the SRVIVR van. I did just fine, too. Until I ran over Pat.

I remember barreling around the corner of the building, a box of lining on my forks, eager to load the waiting semitrailer as fast as I could. I was in a hurry because some of the invoice items had been misplaced, and things were getting backed up. When I rounded the corner of the building, I saw nothing other than a Patless straightaway to the trailer.

Along the edge of the building, in its shadow, just ahead of me and to the left, I saw the two or three towers of wooden palettes stacked under the rooftop overhang. I also saw bright sunlit cement and the bleached gray semitrailer, about thirty yards ahead. But I didn't catch, despite the twenty yards between us, Pat in the shade trying to pull a palette down from the stack, right there in front of me, between the forklift and the trailer. I must have stared at him and the space he occupied for a good five seconds as I sped towards him.

Then an image flashed. He materialized in my eye, just to the left of the forks, a body in contorted motion as he leapt out of the way, safe. Safe and toxic with rage.

Dumb as a lemming, I locked the brakes, and instead of driving ahead, as fast as I could, past the trailer and out of the parking lot, on to 200th street and south for home, or Mexico, or anywhere safe, I stopped to see if he was okay.

"Wow, sorry about that."

Pat flipped his mullet.

"You dick, you did that on purpose!" He stormed towards me. "On purpose! You're fucking dead, Knighton, dead!"

Another lesson in warehouse culture steamrolled my way. Off came Pat's Slack Alice t-shirt. As he picked up speed, his hands balled into fists. He hurled threats and promises of bodily harm, in customary preparation for heavy metal justice. In this kind of trial, court is a loading dock, and arguments are issued in the form of furious pastings. Through drubbings we were meant to reconcile differences or settle old scores. The jury of a few other guys didn't watch in silent judgment. They cheered for blood, anybody's blood.

"No! Pat, no, I didn't. Really—" I pleaded. "It was a mistake, Pat. It was a mistake!"

For added denial, I waved the palms of my hands back and forth in front of me, as if wiping the accident away like a smudge in the air. Pleading only fueled him. He continued to bull my way, a shirtless fury hell bent on punching my clock. Without stopping, he scooped a heavy roll of packing tape from the ground and pitched it. I ducked and heard the sound as the doughnut of tape whizzed over my head.

From inside the semitrailer, Greg must have heard everything. He suddenly shoved me from behind, pushing me aside, and headed straight for Pat with one arm out, hand open like a crossing guard. The gesture, although softly enforced, meant enough to hold Pat in place. Pat raged on the spot. He deeked his face side to side, trying to see around Greg, all the while shooting menacing looks and imploring me to "c'mon, man, c'mon."

"What the hell is going on?" Greg said.

Pat made a show of his answer. "Get outta my way, Greg. I'm warning you, I'm gonna deck this guy."

With a surge of new effort Pat tried to push through but didn't get far. Greg switched fact-finding tactics and put Pat in a headlock.

"Let go, Greg, let go! Bumbleton tried to run me over. Ow, shit, ow."

Greg said he'd let go when Pat calmed down. It took a minute, then Pat's body went sort of limp, his head still nut-crackered like a football in Greg's armpit.

"Knighton, go to the lunchroom," Greg said. "I'll be there in a minute. Pat, you're gonna stay here and cool off. I'm gonna sort this out, and you two are gonna stay apart, and nobody's going to do nothing. Christ, I'm sick of you two."

In the lunchroom I continued to stand my accidental ground.

"It was an accident, Greg, just an accident."

Greg began to make coffee but slammed everything for punctuation—the lunchroom door, the coffee pot on the counter, the old filter into the garbage can. The accident was my fault this time, no dodging it.

"Listen to yourself. Doesn't make sense, Ryan. How the hell do you miss Pat, or anybody, or anything, right there in the middle of a wide open space, and how do you just happen to drive straight for him or it or whatever? Doesn't make any sense to me. You're a klutz, no doubt about it, but nobody, nobody, is that much of a klutz. What you did was just plain stupid."

I didn't know what to say. I didn't have an answer.

Three years and two months later, on my eighteenth birthday, I would learn the truth. An ophthalmologist would tell me I suffer from a degenerative condition known as retinitis pigmentosa. Because of a gene mutation, one I was born with, my retina had begun to scar itself and decay. Little holes were developing in my vision and had been developing for some time. Soon they would expand like blurry pools, band together, and narrow me into the slightest tunnel of sight. Later, perhaps, that last sliver of functional retina would eclipse, too. Either way, I would be legally blind within a few years.

But back in Great West's lunchroom, I didn't know anything about holes in my visual field. I only knew my life had stories and that a few of those had holes in them. Some things couldn't be explained, like the accident with Pat. A person I knew, my sighted self, was disappearing, but I didn't know how or why. To answer Greg, then, and to answer for myself, I defended my bad behaviour the only way I could imagine. I lied.

"I have an eye problem, Greg."

He stopped making coffee. He didn't totally believe me, not yet, but he was curious.

"What kind of eye problem? "

"I have, well, I have this thing, like a spot I can't see through. I, well, I didn't want to tell you because it isn't a big deal, really, it's just sometimes I miss stuff because of it."

It sounded like a reasonable lie. The distinction felt strong enough. My eyes were to blame, but not me. Who would question the diagnosis? Who would know any better?

Greg sprung with new anger, but an anger tinged with regret. "Why the hell didn't you tell me? You should have told me before I let you drive or even work the forks with Pat. For chrissake. You could've fallen or—"

"No, I'm fine, I just—well, I just found out last week, and

the doctor said it was no big deal, really, it's a small thing. Like you said, I have to pay attention. That's all."

He sat down at the lunchroom table and thoughtfully stroked the corners of his moustache. He was no dummy. I'd just about killed someone on his watch, and I was blameless, as only a teenager can be. Generously, he gave me my only chance to repair the damage.

"Be straight with me. I mean it. Are you sure you've got this, this eye problem? I mean, it's okay if it was an accident; accidents happen. Just tell me the truth."

Although we sat across from one another, I couldn't look him in the eye. I fixed my gaze past him, to the pinups on the wall. Miss June's smile mocked me knowingly.

"It's true, Greg. It was an accident."

"Jesus. There's nothing they can do for you?"

A lump of guilt grew in me. I was deceiving someone I admired. I didn't want undeserved sympathy, just an excuse. Underneath it all, I could even feel a smaller but heavier uncertainty—maybe something really was wrong with my eyes. The reality flickered and then was gone. I was fourteen and immortal, part of the new order. Nothing could be wrong, so I supersized my lie.

"No, there's nothing they can do. The damage isn't something they can reverse," I said. "But really, Greg, it's no big thing at all. I'm not getting worse or anything. I just have to pay attention, like you said."

Greg looked both sympathetic and confused.

"But how are you supposed to pay attention to things you don't see?"

From that moment on, his was the question that blindness would demand I answer.

"I don't know," I said. For the first time, I was truthful. "I'll have to figure it out, I guess."

Although I never drove the forklift again, I steered clear of Pat. He didn't give a shit if I was Helen Keller. He didn't believe the forklift incident was an accident. Greg did his best to manage things and reminded Pat of his luck.

"You're a fortunate man," Greg would say. "Bumbleton could've crushed your little legs. Jesus, they're already too cute and stubby to look at."

Greg hired me back the following year. Pat wasn't with the company any more. A few months before I returned to work, grade ten under my belt and my clumsiness on the rise, Pat had delivered a liner and parts to a pool site in Maple Ridge. Backing his van up to the hole, Pat somehow clipped the customer's house and took a chunk for a drive. It was Pat's second major screw-up with backing into things. Greg fired him, and said even Bumbleton can spot a house.

Once I had imagined a summer of fortune for myself. I had hoped the simple difference of my job could race me towards my adulthood, even push me into a world some dead-end McJob could never serve-up. I thought I'd start by driving a forklift, and soon enough I'd be driving out of town for good and ahead with things. It may have been short-sighted at the time, but a future, I thought, could be found in a warehouse. It was true enough.

Instead of wealth, I found another fortune, the kind that is told. Somehow I'd bumbled into my fate as a blind man before it was upon me. The story of my blindness began as a lie. Today I see the fortune I told for myself, and I see it in hindsight. That is nearing the only vision I have left. Maybe Pat's problem was something opposite. He really needed to look back more often, and more thoroughly. Tough luck, I guess. The guy never did get the hang of reverse.

Pontiac Rex

Not seeing something, not seeing an indication of something, does not lead automatically to the conclusion that there is nothing.

   —Hans Blix, *The Guardian*, June 2003

Unbeknownst to my family, my physician, or the motor vehicle branch, by the age of seventeen, I was going blind behind the wheel of my father's 1982 Pontiac Acadian. Feel free to shudder. Other soon-to-be-blind people are on the road today enjoying a similar story, only they've still got some damage to do. Maybe you'll meet one of them at an intersection.

Driving beckoned me the moment I turned sixteen, but my parents thought I'd benefit first from a driver's education course. Or two. Maybe three. I was that hopeless. Not much of what I learned remains in my brain, but I do remember my teacher, a greasy-haired man who insisted I call him Buddy.

For several months, Buddy picked me up once a week in his school's red Ford Taurus. The car was equipped with an extra brake on the passenger side. Buddy liked to punch it through the floor when frightened. Pocked and battered, the car's condition suggested the nifty Siamese brake did little more than relieve the pressure in Buddy's jaw. Nobody could say he was impatient with his students, though, and nobody could say he looked at the world from his car with anything other than safety on his mind. Oh, and ass. A large helping of ass weighed on his mind, too.

When he wasn't advising how to make a generous turn, Buddy gazed out the passenger window, as if avoiding eye contact with his job. Who wouldn't? It probably offered relief from spotting all the gory mishaps I could have steered us into. Some afternoons I could tell that the man was a sack of adrenaline and nerves. As he spoke he'd manically smear his hair across the bald spots on his head. His thoughts flip-flopped at dizzying speeds, all given voice, jumping from death to sex and back again, shaped by a stream of conscious-ness Freud would have enjoyed fishing in. The sidewalks and parking lots we passed provided his material.

"Holy mother of god! Did you see that honey in the elastic jeans? Slow down. The one going into SAAN's back there? What a butt. Jesus that was close! You gotta shoulder check, watch your blind spot. What an a-ass! It makes me—just pull to the right a bit so you don't ride the yellow line. That's right, a little more, don't be afraid of your side of the road. How does she get into those pants? What about blood flow, eh? Signal first! They're like paint."

Sometimes I couldn't tell if Buddy was testing me in his own perverse way. Did his questions measure my awareness? Did the asses tell him if I noticed anything other than the car in front of me? Good drivers, he'd declare, observe every-thing around them. Everything. To underline his point, he'd give an extra wipe of his hair. Sometimes I nodded and muttered something affirmative. I tried to demonstrate that I'd spared some of my abundant driverly attention for the asscape. "Yes, a very different butt from that one back on Fraser Highway, Buddy, quite different." None of this made me a more attentive driver in the end.

Buddy's final report was unambiguous. He recommended another course before I bothered failing the driver's test. It took a lot of practice with my father until my parents felt everybody was safe. Somehow I passed my first road test with only a few demerits, which was unfortunate.

Because of all this I came a year late to driving. My licence, however, which I earned shortly before my seventeenth birthday, came a year earlier than my diagnosis with RP. The math is still chilling. I drove for thirteen danger-filled months, practically blind and legally reckless, unaware of what I was missing. And I mean barely missing.

Before I spill all the gory details, I should explain how it could happen. It's difficult to reconcile how I earned a licence. Some find it hard to believe that a person can be blinded, or slowly blinded, yet remain unaware of the vanishing points. Several explanations are clear to me now.

First, blind spots are not darkness or emptiness in the visual field. Those ideas are in and of themselves visual. Try looking at the floor with your feet. That's what blindness looks like. We can't see it, or see it even as an absence in our experience. An omitted image doesn't alert itself to your attention until, say, you shoot past a stop sign, and, wow, suddenly it appears in the corner of your eye. Only then does it occur to you that something was out there, something that did not appear when it should have. Hard to test for that.

Another explanation is particular to my retinas and their degenerative pattern. Nobody tested me for night vision. An inability to see in the dark is one of the early effects of my disease. When it came to reading the eye chart and identifying the road signs, my eyes did their duty. But put those same signs under a street lamp on a foggy September evening—now that's another phenomenon, and one I would have missed.

I do remember the administrator checking my peripheral vision. He flashed a couple of bright lights to be caught only by the corner of my eye. Fine. Then he checked my central vision with the usual alphabet soup made into an eye chart. I passed that, too. But the real problem was everything else. Imagine your visual field, the dimension of all that you see, shaped like a dart board. I could spot the bull's-eye and the outer ring, but the middle or inner rings, they remained a Swiss cheese of tiny blurs my brain refused to see. My cognition, like anybody's, compensated for the small, missing pockets in between. I saw, in other words, by inferring what wasn't there, what connected the edges to the center of my sight. The holes weren't large, but they were growing, and a lot could disappear within so little. Roll a newspaper and hold it like a telescope to your eye. Huge, distant objects can fit inside. Far enough away, even a truck could drive through. Sometimes they did.

Finally, nobody tested for the depth perception I didn't have. Had the administrator of my exam seen me on the job, now waiting tables in a local café, he may have thought twice about taking my picture and giving me a licence to cruise. At work, my hands regularly jammed through stands of water glasses when I meant to grab the first one. Dropping plates on a table with excessive force, as if in disgust at a customer's preference for blue cheese dressing over a nice balsamic, was a habit, too. Like my days at the pool factory, these manners were dismissed as traits of my character. Ryan, the clumsy guy who slams things. So moody, so distracted.

Sure, I sensed difficulty when I drove, but it came and went depending on the weather or time of day. Driving home at night from the café, the roads dark and wet with rain, I could vaguely detect the double yellow line. I thought, as my parents had said, the problem was my lack of experience. They also agreed it could be difficult to spot a painted line on a puddled street. What did I know? I wasn't going to dispute my parents' opinion or insist my difficulties were a tad worse than they imagined. Argue myself out of driving? I was seventeen, not some kind of safety nut. To help find the rainy night lines, I often relied on the raised cat's eyes, the solid reflectors that peppered most of the routes home. Not that I looked at them. If no other cars could help me position myself in my lane, I'd ride the cat's eyes and feel for the "clunk clunk clunk" under my tires. At night I drove Braille. Didn't everybody?

I kept the first accident to myself. The very afternoon I pocketed my driver's licence, I drove straight to my girl-friend's house to take her out for a spin and anything else a car might encourage. She wasn't home. As I left the winding streets of her neighbourhood, I fumbled with all the serious business of driving. I lit a smoke, or tried to, fast-forwarded a

Smiths tape I'd just bought, stopped and started the cassette player, listened for that Johnny Marr riff I liked, steered and clutched and shifted gears, and with the successfully tested corner of my eye, caught a stop sign as I sailed past.

The red shape flashed, disappeared from view, and then lit in me the sharp recognition that I was about to meet some kind of consequence, probably a loud and painful type. The view immediately brightened. The periphery of the narrow, residential street opened up, as did the surprised expression on my face. Fast-moving cars surrounded me, all of them motoring at a right angle to my own. I was about to spear the panel of a cube van, two cars were about to t-bone the driver's side of mine, and some other vehicles, the ones out my passenger window, looked like they were fleeing the scene. All I could do was watch in horror and awe as I rocketed across four lanes of traffic.

What to do? Brake? Speed up? Combinations? Time lingers more than it should in circumstances like this. It hung around in my car, making more of itself, piling on, the feeling of its dead weight slowing me down, drawing out the drama of expectation and allowing me to witness each potential calamity in slow motion until, eventually, I arrived on the other side, astonished and safe.

Not one car had careened or locked its brakes as I'd crossed the street. Not one car had touched another car. Not a single person had been hurt. It must have looked beautiful from the sidewalk, as if I'd divined a pause, a perfect rest in the busy traffic, then cut through, effortless and smooth. A fish in a stream.

I wanted to puke. Immediately I pulled over and parked on the side of the road until the panic and nausea dissolved. What was I supposed to do now? Emergency lights, I thought, that's what they're called, emergency lights. I flicked them on. They didn't help. I got out and ran back to the intersection to look for what I'd done. It was daft, but something in me wanted to see if my accident left some kind of trace. Not a thing remained. Cars slipped by in their usual way and the stop sign across the street declared what I should have done. Nobody waited to chastise me. Nobody demanded I apologize. It was as if the accident had never happened. So I took my cue and agreed to keep it that way. A promise was made, instead, a promise to be more careful, to be less hasty, to be focused, to be happy with whatever song is playing in my cassette deck. Back into the car I climbed, turned off the emergency lights, and pulled away, nonchalant as a poacher with his catch.

My second accident happened some months later. It even earned me a title. All hail the Rock King of Langley.

The few dwindling back roads of my hometown are darkened by thick stands of trees. When I was a teenager, you wouldn't find much out there other than turkey farms, Christmas tree nurseries, houses set far into their fields, and the occasional business that surprised the side of the road with a few muddy parking spots. You might find a decaying John Deere dealership out there and a forgotten TV repair shop from the 1950s. That's about it. Gas stations were the only other oasis of light I remember seeing on a night drive. Like a good son should, I had just topped up my father's tank at one of those gas stations before I ascended my throne.

Leaving the station, I nosed the car to the edge of the road and checked for oncoming traffic. Black to the left, black to the right. The country road was moonlit and empty. I flicked my turn signal on and dumped the clutch. The engine accelerated, its hum grew louder, then an alien crunch and grind overtook my ears. Up went the car. The front popped a wheelie and dropped, as if the Acadian had pounced on some massive, unsuspecting prey. I wasn't moving anymore.

From my strange new perspective, I stared up at the clear evening sky instead of down the clear, open road. I took a quiet moment to tally how many un-good things had just transpired. When I turned the key, the car started again. I surged with relief. But easing forward wasn't easy. It wasn't even possible. The car sputtered and stalled. Down in front, little revealed itself other than what I thought was the road I should be driving home. What I'd heard and seen didn't make sense, so I got out, and my first step took more leg than usual.

What I'd taken to be the road wasn't the road at all. Under my feet I felt a nice patch of lawn that I'd turned the car on to. More worrisome, though, I'd made it almost halfway over a line of large, decorative boulders. My car—my father's car— had impaled itself on one. Now, together, rock and vehicle made something like a Pontiac lean-to. Stonehenge, I thought.

My Stonehenge had its tourists, too. Their eyes watched me from inside the gas station's store. Nobody approached, though, and nobody seemed interested in offering me some engineering advice. Maybe the two gas jockeys hadn't noticed what I'd done to their lawn, after all. Either way, I wanted out of my embarrassment as fast as possible. Damages shmamages, if it took a little more grinding to get the job done.

I climbed back in, which is to say I climbed back up, and put the car into neutral. My hope was that the car might slide off the rock. Reptiles and dead things always slid off rocks on those animal documentaries. The Acadian didn't give. I got out and tried to push, but it still wasn't going anywhere. A voice called from the gas station's door. One of the two jockeys.

"Hey, man! Are you, like, stuck or something?"

"No, I'm just fine," I shouted back. I waved, too, the way people do when they pass on pleasure boats. I thought the affectation would deter him. Long, long way to go if you want to walk over here. Got to wave, it's so far. "There's no problem," I said. "I'm just, I'm just checking something."

I hopped up into the car again. I had to leave, no matter what. How would I explain to my parents that I was perched on a stone about ten feet shy of the turn? I started the engine, put the car in gear, and fed it all the gas I could. The tires spun, caught, and set off a fantastic noise as I launched from the rock and landed on the lawn in front of it. Now, instead of crucified on a boulder, I was safe and level. Sort of.

A new challenge revealed itself. Had I looked harder, I might have noticed the lawn wasn't simply edged by boulders, but encircled by them. My father's car was free, and in the middle.

I got out and tried to look confident. I was a man with a plan, a stranded-car plan. This time a different voice called from the gas station.

"That's much better! Good for you!"

Over the car's roof I could see the two jeering gas jockeys silhouetted in the store's doorway.

"That's it, I'm gonna call Clover Towing," the first voice said. "Don't do anything. I'll get a tow truck to . . . I dunno, lift you or something."

"No," I called back. "It's all fine! I'm just . . . leaving. See you later. Thanks anyway."

I was uncertain what to do other than go. I put the car in gear, aimed for the smallest big rock, and gunned for it. The anticipated noise erupted underneath. The car lifted and dropped on a slant as I humped over the wall and back into the gas station's tiny parking lot, a couple of decorative boulders rolling after me, a few feet from their craters.

"Very good thinking!" The cheerleading gas guy could barely contain himself. "You are a smart one, aren't you."

His colleague was less impressed. "You stupid fuckhead!" he shouted. "You big fucking fuckhead!"

I nosed the car to the edge of the road. When I found it for sure, I lit my turn signal for the gas jockeys, and sped away. The word "fuckhead" floated in my open window one more time, so I gave a couple toots on the horn.

I intended to keep the story to myself, but the light of day didn't help. The next morning my father left the house for work. A few minutes later, his heavy boots stomped back into the kitchen. Oil covered his hands and wrists like a pair of evening gloves. I continued to shovel cereal into my mouth and pretended not to notice him. Standing at the sink, he lathered his hands and broke the silence.

"So, it seems we have a bit of an oil leak out there."

I didn't look up from reading the cereal box. "Really?" I said. "Well, I guess the Acadian is getting old."

"How do you know I'm not talking about your mother's car?"

I chewed and pretended I could only hear my crispy cereal.

"Put your shoes on and we'll have a look together. You'll learn something." He paused for added effect and dried his hands on a tea towel. "Maybe I'll learn something, too."

My parents were a mighty talent at that sort of threat. They never directly chewed us out. First they tossed a line, one that told us something was coming, something swift, inevitable, and just. They'd let us feel the pressure in the room change and let us stew in the vacuum. Usually it was enough to pull the confessions loose.

I knew I was nailed, but I made it out of the kitchen without giving in to any wrongdoing. I hoped that my performance could outlive Dad's suspicions. We stood beside the car for a moment, then he motioned for me to have a look underneath. The street appeared to have dissolved into a pond of oil.

"Wow," I said. "How'd you notice that?"

"Funny thing, see the metal there under the door and all along the side?"

The bottom of the car no longer held a smooth line. It

looked like the lip of a clam shell. "I noticed that first and then the oil."

"Yeah, I guess it's kind of hard to miss."

"Uh huh."

Dad fixed his expression. As I spoke, he looked at me as if waiting for me to finish something I wanted to say.

"Guess that's quite a bit of work fixing a bad leak like that."

"Uh huh."

"Goddamn cars, eh? Always something to fix."

"Uh huh."

"Say, who do you think is the best mechanic in Langley?"

He didn't answer.

"The best besides you, I mean."

"You know, Ryan, it's a funny thing. The car wasn't like that yesterday. Today it leaks oil, and yesterday it didn't. Call me crazy, but I'm thinking last night something happened? You would be the last person in the car, too, so I'm thinking . . ."

I copped to it before he outright stated, in no uncertain terms, it was my fault. Better to admit it than to hear the blame. But the making of Stonehenge turned out to be a difficult phenomenon to describe.

"Rocks?" my father scowled. "Explain this to me again. Where did you find these rocks?"

"I didn't find them. They were just there."

His scowl deepened. "And how exactly did you get my car on top of them?"

Again I described how, in the dark, the patch of lawn had looked like the road I tried to leave by, and how the rocks weren't there, but then they were.

"Of course," he said. A big smile broke under his big moustache. "Of course it was the grass, the grass that looked like a road."

"Right."

"And it was the wall of rocks."

"Right."

"The ones you missed."

"Yes."

"But then found underneath the car."

He didn't believe a word of it.

At dinner that night, one of my younger brothers, Rory, asked if I could drive him somewhere. He probably didn't have anywhere pressing to be, really, being twelve, but the two of us liked to go out in Dad's car, buy junk food, and goof around. Rory was a nervous kid, a bit of a loner, and I liked taking him out with me. The first time I drove him somewhere, I asked if he wanted to shift the gears. He looked at me with disbelief, like I'd offered him my bank account.

"Really? You're gonna let me change gears?" he asked. "But I don't know how."

"I'll tell you which gear and when. Maybe I'll let you steer a little, too, If you want."

His face told me that I was now more than his older brother. I was Santa Claus, and perhaps superhuman. Then his nervousness overtook him, as it always did. "But what if we get in an accident?" he said.

"Jesus, would you relax? We won't get in an accident. I'll be in control. I'm trying to offer you some fun here. Don't be such a suck."

"I'm not being a suck. I just don't wanna get in trouble."

"That's why you're a suck. We're supposed to get in trouble sometimes. I'm your big brother. I'm supposed to teach you this kind of stuff. Relax, for chrissake."

With Dad's car I'd tried to become the older brother I'd always wanted, the one who taught his kid brother how to smoke, light a bottle rocket, and drive a stick-shift. Sharing the car with Rory quickly built that kind of trust and friendship between us. We started to become real brothers there.

After that, Rory always wanted a lift somewhere. This time, when he asked at dinner for a ride, my mother informed him that the Rock King would be on foot for a while.

"Who's the Rock King?" Rory asked.

My father pointed his fork at me but didn't explain my new title.

Rory found it hilarious. "Ryan is the Rock King," he sang, "king of the rocks, the one who rocks out on top!" He wanked on an air guitar, repeating my new name, and made pouty, guitar-solo faces.

The name stuck for weeks and ridiculed my story. I heard the doubt. My excuse sounded like a cartoon to my parents. Today they insist they believed me, but today I'm a blind guy whose diagnosis made sense of the rocks that punched a hole under the driver's seat, among other things. Holes in the eyes, holes in the car, and more holes in the stories.

From that moment on, I wasn't allowed to drive my father's car at night, not until, he said, I was a more experienced driver. As it turned out, I would only drive a car once more in the dark. That's when I crashed for the last time.

Most accidents might not have given away my growing blindness. They would look too much like accidents other people could have. A missed sign, a poorly judged turn, a distracted change of lanes, too much speed. My final accident had a character unto itself, though, one that we couldn't name clumsiness or inexperience. Speed was a factor, but not in a way anyone could understand.

I remember the sound of my mother marching down the hall to find out what my father and I were arguing about. At three o'clock in the morning, most debates a seventeen-year-old boy could be having with his father won't be going very far. Mine was no exception. My girlfriend was waiting outside on the porch, which didn't help my chances.

"But she's lost her keys," I explained, "and nobody's home, or at least nobody answered when she rang the bell a few times. She can't just sleep on the lawn, right? So I said she should walk home with me and stay overnight here. I thought you'd be cool about it." Some sarcasm, I felt, might add colour here. "But I guess turning her out will be better."

Dad didn't flinch. I braved one more shot.

"I guess I was wrong to think you'd understand."

As the words left my mouth, I saw their stupidity and waste. My parents never took well to passive aggression. They gave more consideration to junk mail.

"Yes," my father snapped, "you were wrong. At least you got something right. And, by the way, I actually do understand. I understand you want your girlfriend to stay over-night, and I also understand that she's not going to stay."

"Who's staying over?" my mother asked as she stepped into the kitchen, tying her robe around her small, intimidating frame.

Over the years, Ma has worked as a psychiatric nurse, a cellblock matron at the local cop shop, and a 911 dispatcher. Her cheerful character often suited her cheerless jobs. She is observant, decisive, fair, and jackboot tough. Together, all five feet and change of my mother has the presence of a razor. It cut away any hope that Karen would be spending the night. The story about lost keys was true, but, admittedly, I'd marked it for a good pretense to have Karen over. Ma would see that, no doubt. I turned back to my father for refuge.

"Well, what do you think I should do, then?" I asked. I hoped he would be stumped for an answer.

"Let's see. Hmm, I know. You take the keys, you drive her home, and you take a screwdriver to open a window."

"Fine," I conceded.

"Have you been drinking?"

My parents knew we'd been at a party. I knew something different. A dozen of us had actually been hard at work helping our friend Andrew harvest any magic mushrooms we could find around his family farm. I hadn't eaten any this time, but Karen, I imagined, was having a wonderful visit with our front porch.

"No," I lied. "I didn't drink anything." Three beers didn't seem to be enough to get in even more trouble over.

Karen's bedroom window was unlocked, after all. Getting

her inside didn't prove to be much of a problem. Only the mushrooms got in the way.

"Windows are cool," she informed me.

I held her up by the feet and tried to help her through. Karen seemed to forget the purpose of standing there, opting to gawk instead of move.

"I'm, like, all about windows. I'm so pro-windows," she said, then climbed in for the night.

I couldn't linger. I knew my father would be waiting up for me, so I drove straight home, careful to stop at the end of Karen's street when the sign told me to.

It was early September and unseasonably cold. Fog crowded its way into the lower stretches of the route home and made it hard for me to see my turn. I could make out the streetlights, but the fog smeared the lights across my eyes, wiping out anything the brightness intended to catch. A car approached. Its headlights burst in the fog and made an obstacle I couldn't see around. I slowed down and dropped the car into first gear, barely inching along the road, and listened to the other car speed past. How could it do that? None approached from behind, and none approached in front. I was alone and creeping in the dark, the closest thing I could manage to feeling my way home with my functional four senses trapped inside the car. I wanted to turn the headlights sideways to light the periphery. The best I could do was guess where to turn.

When I judged I was close, even in the middle of the intersection, I cranked to the right. It wasn't the road, though, and it wasn't a grassy patch. This time I felt the car lean and slowly descend into a ditch. Calm, as if used to this sort of thing, I braked and turned off the car. I hadn't crashed. I had, essentially, parked Dad's car on the bank.

When I tried to back out, the tires were helpless against the wet grass. Instead of retreating, I slid a bit further down. My father had just installed a cell phone in his car that week, the newest thing going. I tried it out for the first time. The receiver was so large it felt like a VHS tape against my ear. At home the phone rang, and I almost hoped nobody would answer.

In the headlights of my mother's car, I could better appreciate what I'd done. Dad's car was a foot or so shy of the water at the very bottom of the ditch but fully parked on one side of the deep embankment. The car looked out of place but oddly peaceful, too. Kind of sleepy. No hint of violence or high-speed trauma could be read into it. Dad walked around the scene, inspected for tire rubber on the road, dents in the fender, anything to explain how this could have happened, but no damage and no evidence of reckless speeding could be found. Another fifteen feet and I would've made the turn.

"I wasn't speeding. I turned, and I guess I missed the road," I repeated. I couldn't offer anything more than the self-evident.

"I can see that, Ryan."

When my father makes a sentence, it's never good to hear your name at the end of it. Dad dragged on his cigarette, exhaled hard through his nose, and chased the smoke with his signature, heavy sigh. The arc of my life readied for its final descent. When my father sighs, he sounds like a bull saddened by the colour red.

"Honestly, I couldn't see the turn."

"Do—you—see—it—now?" he boomed.

"Yes, but that's because the extra lights are on. Mom's car makes it—"

"Don't split hairs, Ryan. If you can see what you've done, you can see enough to . . . to not have done it!"

He looked down the road and saw the tow truck coming. I heard its diesel engine.

"How am I to understand this, Ryan? Did you fall asleep? Were you driving the shoulder?" I didn't answer. "Are you drunk?"

I worried I could still have beer breath and didn't want to have that offense on my head, as well.

"Okay, I had two or three beers at the party, but that was hours ago and I'm not drunk at all," I pleaded. "I just . . . I didn't . . ."

Nothing more could be argued. He'd found his answer to the slow wreck. That was enough. Dad paid to have the car towed home instead of letting me drive it.

For two excruciating days, my father refused to speak to me. When I walked in a room, he left. If I asked him to pass the beans, he did, but put them down with a slam. I was with Greg in the lunchroom all over again. Yes or no questions were given nods or grunts. Ma carried on, business as usual, but her chipper edge had dulled. Quietly, she made an appointment to have my eyes checked, just in case, but stayed out of the situation, otherwise. Like me, I suspect she also waited for dad to break. Even my brothers and sisters waited, mostly in their rooms, like animals sensing a nasty shift in weather. Then, one afternoon when he was driving me home from work, he suddenly pulled over and put on the emergency lights.

He turned to me and broke into a fury I've never known since. It was like rocketing across four lanes of traffic, every horn honking and every tire squealing. The emergency lights ticked their beat, but I could feel time slowing down, as it does.

In his rage my father surveyed everything I'd done to endanger myself. I'd lied about drinking. I'd lied about not seeing the turn in order to hide the fact that I'd been drinking, and who knows if I'd done this before. He'd clearly reconsidered the legend of the Rock King. Then he reminded me about my mother's job at the police station, what she sees and hears every day about drunk drivers. I'd endangered myself, my family, strangers, and in his judgment, I'd demonstrated unforgivable idiocy. The only thing I had going for me was luck. I was lucky, he said, that's all, and being lucky doesn't make it any better.

We sat in silence on the side of the road. Soaked in self-pity, I stared out the window for an answer and fidgeted with loose change in my cup holder. Dad lit a cigarette and resumed not looking at me. My only option was a confession. At least I could fill in the missing cause with apology. So I did. I apologized for driving drunk. I swore I would never do it again. My tone had all the sincerity I could find but still rang empty to me. Just a prop to stand in for whatever the truth really was.

When he finished his cigarette, Dad flicked the butt out the window and said it would be a long time before he trusted me again. I had to earn it back. How or if I could do that wasn't clear to him. He turned the emergency lights off, and we pulled away. We never spoke about the accident again.

Within a week or two the calm returned between us, but something was missing. Dad could feel it, too. The first casualty of distrust, I learned, is familiarity. My father saw me as a slightly different person now. Part of me was a stranger to him. Since my time at Great West Pool, that seed of estrangement had grown in me, too. More than ever, I didn't know how to account for the gap between my intentions and my mistakes.

So many tales of blindness return to the subject of guilt. I think of Oedipus unable to look at what he'd done, or what some would say he was fated to do. But it was an accident, and I'm confident that's why he took his eyes. Fate is blameless and much easier to look upon than anything one can regret. To believe fate made him do it would've saved Oedipus a lot of grief. When it came to my car accident, to know blindness made me do it would've saved both my father and me a lot of grief, too.

In a way, both Oedipus and I destroyed our fathers while travelling the road home. The car accident was my fault, no doubt, but when my family and I learned later that I was going blind, my failing eyesight confused the ownership of all that blame. It wasn't my fault anymore. The guilt became my father's, instead.

Like other diseases, I suspect, one peculiar misfortune of my own is its lack of boundaries. Blindness doesn't keep its consequences within my skin. It crashes into the lives of others, family, friends, and strangers, and transforms those lives as well. My father was my first victim. From me he still takes upon himself a regret for what I did that night in his car. It's guilt for his assumption that I'd lied about what I could and couldn't see, and for chastising his blind son. I wasn't drunk, I was blind, and he hadn't trusted me. I know he's never forgiven himself. I don't know how to relieve him of the guilt, either. In that lies the real accident and the real heartbreak. I just can't keep blindness to myself.

The afternoon we drove home from the eye doctor's office, having just learned that I was going blind, my father and I passed the ditch. I looked at the spot, not having thought about it for some time. I felt a unique relief. Something strange in my past, something I couldn't account for, finally belonged to me, and made sense, even. It's true good drivers notice everything. I know my father looked at that ditch, too, and recognized, for the first time, what had really happened. My stories were becoming true. We didn't talk about the ditch and the accident, though. We let it pass. Only a few blocks remained before we'd be home. Ma was there preparing my eighteenth birthday dinner. She would be the next person I couldn't keep my blindness from.

My diagnosis still hadn't sunk in, not really, yet I felt unbearably anxious. I didn't want to tell my mother that we'd learned I'd be blind within a matter of years. It would kill her. I had no choice, though, no way out. My diagnosis was going to hurt her, and I didn't know how to do that.

When we arrived home, Dad and I took our shoes off at the front door. His hand motioned for me to go downstairs to my room. I headed down but stopped at the bottom of the stairwell to listen. My mother was up in the kitchen with my brothers and sister, peeling potatoes and making salads for my birthday party. She asked Dad how things went at the doctor's office.

He walked into the kitchen and told my brothers and sister to go outside for awhile. When they were gone, he sat down at the table with Ma and poured them both a coffee. I couldn't hear everything they said, but I didn't have to. I knew my father was about to hurt my mother for me, and then he did.

At Home with Punk

Night blindness, or moon blindness, is easily misunderstood. It doesn't only mean someone sees jack-squat when the lights go out. Even a little light can be too little. Many folks in my condition are blinkered by ambient restaurants, while others experience night blindness in the slanted rays of dusk, and all of us, well, we take a moonlit stroll and we know too well black is black. Shades of night blindness abound, which can make the condition unapparent to us all, the night blind included. Hell, when it first came upon me, I couldn't spot my own night blindness if you'd lit it on fire and handed me some gas in a spritzer bottle.

Within a year of my diagnosis, I became totally night blind. That completed the first stage of my retinal deterioration, according to my doctor, and thus indicated the ready onset of further degeneration in my peripheral vision and central acuity, blah blah blah. Who the hell cares, I thought. Certainly not me, not at the time. Not with that nineteen-year-old hormone festival in my body. I felt I had more pressing concerns than some rumoured future of blindness. Moving out on my own, for instance, would be neat.

Instead of listening to my doctor, I shrugged off the details and, as much as possible, nursed disinterest in my so-called medical decline. Except for one thing. Armed with a teen savvy for self-serving opportunism, I used night blindness as doctor's orders to get out of Dodge. The pitch to my parents went something like this: "I can't live at home anymore, Ma, I gotta go—you know—before I can't see." I figured my parents could use the room, anyway. We lived in a boxy house stuffed with four kids and a lot of pets. The time was right to strike out on my own. Because I was night blind, though, most things in the world would strike me first.

Night blindness changed my body, but it also changed my place in the world. It permanently coloured my relationship to the suburbs, for one thing. My new body, in time, grew intolerant, even hostile, to the useless, long suburban side-walks and their grid. I couldn't travel them well anymore, either on foot by day or, now, by any means in the dark. No doubt my childhood streets were great for ball hockey and BMX bikes, but they weren't amenable to young men who can't steer clear of a ditch. The urban planners hadn't antici-pated odd physiologies like mine. Buses in Langley were infrequent and erratic. I knew where I wasn't wanted. I took the hint. Gladly, in fact.

My parents, always supportive, didn't really need my excuse to help me do whatever I saw fit. I'd completed enough college courses to obliterate my high school grades, a chronicle of my early loafing, and was ready to transfer to a local university. Before those first classes began, I moved out, with a truckload of donated rattan furniture and a mound of aging appliances and kitchenware, all of which my folks had scrounged from coworkers and friends. Dad strapped the works down on a one-ton flat deck and used my pillows to keep the ropes from cutting into the edges of IKEA bookcases and my mother's ancient brown easy chair, my favourite, the velour one. Finally we backed out of the driveway, and I left home. My moving truck looked like an inheritance from the Beverly Hillbillies. I have yet to meet someone whose first kitchen had two cake decorating sets, as mine did. Such are my parents and their unbridled generosity.

My new roommate, Jane, was a deaf student also attending Simon Fraser University. Yes, deaf. This, our poetry courses would teach us, was poetic. She was slender and sweet, spoke with a slight lisp, and wore hearing aids, unless she didn't want to hear anything or anybody, which was most of the time. Jane's most notable feature, however, was her hair. She cared for a long mane of the bushiest, curliest tendrils I've ever seen, hair so big and poofed that Jane could only paint it down with tubs of salon goo. Nothing really worked, though. In short, she was a terrific character who misread my lips daily. Jane also happened to be the daughter of some church buddies my grandparents favoured. She was looking for a roommate at the same time as me. We'd never met before. We weren't friends, not yet, but we shared a need to transplant ourselves out of our homes and closer to school. Everything seemed to be mutually beneficial. Even perfect.

We were the true Odd Couple, and it helped. Being in the company of the other's disability was a comfort of sorts. Our denial, or struggle, or whatever attitude we took to our fucked-up bodies on any given day, gave us each some private reassurance, when we didn't see an apartment full of the

other person's fear. Mostly the absurdity of our match
amused us.

"Hi, you've reached the answering machine for Ryan and
Jane. We're probably home right now, but Jane didn't hear
the phone again, and I can't find it. Please leave a message.
Or just come over and help."

Our bodies weren't as poorly designed as our new apartment. The ugly digs Jane and I chose were irredeemably
close to our new school. You may be familiar with Simon
Fraser University. It's the depressing concrete monolith that
often doubles for the Pentagon in movies and *The X-Files*.
The university's architecture is that oppressive, and because
it sits on top of a mountain, in the clouds that rain on
Vancouver, the architecture is forever wet. We lived as close
as we could.

It seemed wise at the time, in the practical and dull sense of
wise. The goal was to minimize bus trips after evening classes
and to diminish my potential for getting lost among the darkened shrubberies of low-cost apartment blocks. Proximity
validated my excuse for moving out, not that I really needed
one. I didn't believe a word of my rationale, really. Like any
respectable nineteen-year-old, I just didn't want to listen to
my parents' music anymore. Where I lived didn't matter to
me at all, as long as I had the keys to let the people and par-
ties come and go. What I hadn't considered, though, was the
holy trinity of fun: location, location, location.

Not to exaggerate, but the neighbourhood and apartment
we chose sucked, and sucked beyond any definition of
sucked I'd known. My life was deeply suburban all over

again, deeply boring, deeply in service of long television nights and delivered pizzas. That I had chosen this place made it all the worse, as if I'd doomed myself to some version of Langley forever. I was becoming the Sisyphus of the cul-de-sacs. Today I think of that time near SFU as the year of brown carpets, soupy smelling hallways, rented movies, and a suppressed fear of going out in the dark. Nothing chained me to my second-hand sofa, but I'd imprisoned myself in order to avoid a life that would reveal my blindness to me in all its force and difficulty. As long as I stayed home, I was okay, and okay meant living in a state of self-loathing with *M*A*S*H* reruns lighting the room. But I still didn't think of myself as a blind guy. Not at all, not yet.

I found it hard to understand or even believe I was night blind. Bullshit, I thought, I can't be night blind yet. I can still stand on my deck at midnight, count the streetlights, and see the tip of my burning cigarette. Even a star or two was visible if I bothered to look up and indulge my neglected awe for the cosmos. I found night blindness difficult to identify or accept because I could see light, be it candlelight, flashlight, or, soon to become my favourite, strobe light. But I failed to spot anything those lights intended to brighten, unless the lights were very intense. A lava lamp in my room, I could see that, but it floated like the sun itself, supported by nothing, suspended from nothing, just a ball of oozy luminescence surrounded by a great deal of space. Isn't that what everybody saw? Isn't that why we invented fluorescent tubes? Night blindness can be, in fact, a lot like a night sky. Visible points of light are here and there, the ones we might wish upon, and a whole lot of vaporous mystery stretches between them. Often I tripped over the vaporous mysteries in my room as I fumbled my way to the light switch or headed for the door in search of bigger city lights and brighter city kicks. I needed to look beyond the black hole of the suburbs and find a suitable place for my pathology. And I did, kind of.

It took some courage and willpower to tackle the evening streets of downtown Vancouver, but eventually I found its nightclubs, as well as my desire for them. Four, sometimes five nights a week, as many as I could withstand, I began to brave my way into the downtown core. There I looked for the scenes and people I had always wanted to become a part of, the ones that never visited me on Beaverbrook Crescent while Jane sewed and I stared blankly out our living-room window.

You might think an appetite for something called a night-club would be a bad idea for someone called night blind. You would be right. Equally wise would be me joining a gun club. Nevertheless, to this day I owe a debt to punk rock. Its culture helped me become as blind as I was but couldn't admit to being.

My apprenticeship into the club scene had numerous dangers and disadvantages, although most were silly. In my time I have argued with empty bar stools, talked to pillars, knocked down waitresses, bounced off bouncers, pissed between urinals, drunk other people's beers, and hit on shadows. Even though I routinely tumbled down stairs and plummeted off stages, never, not once, did it convince me to perhaps take up a white cane. Bullshit, I thought. I'm not that night blind. I'm just drunk.

When the coloured strobes and spotlights did their job, pulsing and spinning with the music, then I was more or less able to see enough. Stepping off the dance floor into the murky bar, that was a bit of a problem. Slow songs, too. They always dropped the lights down for slow songs, which left me paralysed wherever I happened to be. For a moment, anyway. Then like a jerky Sex Pistol I'd career off the dance floor, knocking people over instead of politely scooting around them. I was a poser, not nearly close to hardcore, but blindness lent an authenticity to my recklessness. I ignored every social propriety our eyes manage.

That was the best thing about the scene. The culture camouflaged my inability to cooperate with other bodies. In growing blindness I became, oddly enough, safer and more like the postpunk scenesters around me than I was like my peers at school. Booze helped. Everybody was bent, legless, gassed, rat-arsed, and every other word for blind drunk. Bumping into people was acceptable, even expected, and I was practised at bashing into folks on a regular basis, whether I was in my cups or just spilling them. Confusion and disorientation ruled the clubs, too, and that pretty much described my sober state. Above all, though, I blended with ease and advantage on the dance floor. I loved to slam. What blind person doesn't?

When the opening bars of a thrashy song burst from the sound system, I felt in my muscles my own rhythm of relief. Here I could be a blind man and feel it, or test it, for a while. Somebody's elbow would clock me in the face, and we were off. Up and down we jumped and flung ourselves aimlessly in any direction, a random application of weight, speed, shoulders, fists, heads, and boots, all hoping to meet another body, sandwich a few, or sometimes miss altogether and drop ourselves. A ragged enthusiasm. Family fun. But in all that I was relaxed and abandoned, a pro at the art of whacking and rebounding, while some could never give themselves completely over. Many tried too hard to control themselves, tried to brace and aim, as if they could do that. Dumb. In the middle of a slam, or a mosh pit, or whatever it's called now, abandon is the key to survival and pleasure. You can't predict what's coming. You can't aim at a moving crowd. You should shut your eyes and go. In my case, I left them open. I loved to slam. It was where my blindness worked. It was the antidote to where I lived, be it behind my failing eyes or behind my nervous, suburban door.

Then I began to lose things other than my eyesight.

It started at a gig at the Commodore Ballroom, one of Vancouver's oldest venues and one of its finest. Rubber tires supported the old wooden dance floor. A crowd could easily get a good trampoline effect going. One night somebody stepped on my heel and off my shoe popped. It was gone, kicked about like a soccer ball, boinking across the floor. I chased after it but didn't get very far. Mostly I stared down in disbelief at my sock, which I couldn't quite make out, either. My friend Peter spotted my shoe. It was briefly in the air and travelling in the general direction of the stage. Looked like trouble for the bass player. According to Peter, my shoe connected with her head. Without losing a beat, she booted my Doc Marten off stage, into the wings. I had to wait until the show was over and the club was clearing out until a roadie agreed to go shoe hunting backstage. Twenty bucks to get it back. I was proud. The bass player for Lush had touched my shoe with her face.

I should have taken this as a sign that slamming in nightclubs was not the best of hobbies, but my evening schedule was too busy for reflection. Not one week passed before Peter and I found ourselves in a different club. This time somebody knocked the glasses off my face. They dropped to the floor like a hockey puck, and the chase was on, once again. Peter went after my specs, his body hunched over and scurrying about the floor like a man chasing a renegade pet. Somehow he snagged my glasses from the trampling herd, and somehow the frames had survived. Not even the slightest bend or lightest scratch. I put my glasses back on, and, presto, I still couldn't see very much. All was right. I was touched by the Slam Gods, clearly.

So it seemed, until I lost my pants.

I adored those pants as much as pants can be reasonably adored. They were polyester and vertically striped, black, green, and grey, and they flared at the ankles. One of my younger brothers, Mykol, who was at the club with me that night, called them my Jack Tripper trousers. He said *Three's Company* was about as retro as one could go without dressing Amish. The only trouble was my pants fit a bit too snuggly in the waist. A complex zipper system inside the belt line kept them tight, a system which I'd let out to its fullest, but still my pants remained a little more constricting than when I'd bought them. The likely cause was all the beer and burgers

I'd begun to live on, as well as the bags of leftover chocolate cream cheese muffins Jane brought home after her shifts at Muffin Inn. Like my attitude toward night blindness, I denied my growing belly and figured I'd dance my way around it.

Then, one night somebody thumped me good in the belly during a Ramones tune, forcing me to double over. The force split the zipper system from its outer limits. My size 33 pants ballooned to a size 45 or so. When I stood up straight, they dropped to my ankles. Immediately I pulled them up and jammed my hands in my pockets. That's how I remained as I shuffled my way to the can to find out what the hell was going on.

It's not the proudest moment in a young man's life when he is standing in a public washroom in his underwear and combat boots, holding his pants up to the light as if inspecting holiday slides. It didn't take me long to admit defeat. I couldn't see much with the little light available, and I obviously knew more about nineteenth-century verse than the engineering and repair of zippers. Back I climbed into my pants, and back my hands went into my pockets. I left the can in search of my brother.

I found him after a couple of revealing circuits around the club. In that short time, shuffling about with my hands in my pockets, my night blindness became more apparent to me than ever before. My fingers weren't available to touch the edges of tables, or to find the railings of staircases. Moving about like a blind amputee, the darkness in me bloomed, even deepened, and suddenly, without hands to help me, I felt how much compensation I'd grown accustomed to. I felt it missing in my fingers like a phantom itch.

When I spotted Mykol, he was near the bar, under an ultraviolet light that illuminated his white cowboy shirt. I could barely make out the shadow of embroidered guns on his shoulders. Mykol has no shortage of fashion irony. Lucky for me, it made him easy to spy. And where would an underage kid be other than at the bar?

"I need to borrow your eyes," I said.

"Sure. What do you need?"

"I need you to come to the bathroom with me."

"No, thanks," Mykol said. "Feel free to watch yourself in there."

"No, no, it's my pants," I explained. "My pants are broken."

Mykol paused and sipped his drink. I heard myself and what I was saying.

"Broken pants?" he asked. "You have broken pants? Who breaks their pants? I don't have a sewing kit, if that's what you need."

"Just come with me and you'll see," I said. "Please. Like, now."

Mykol could hear the urgency in my voice, so he dropped the banter and walked ahead, towards the bathroom. We hadn't walked far before he sensed my trouble with following him. He stopped and extended his elbow to me for guidance. Mykol was always good at knowing when I could see and when I couldn't. I wanted the elbow, but I didn't have a hand available.

"I can't," I yelled above the music. "If I take my hands out of my pockets, my pants will drop."

Without a word or a snicker, he moved behind me and pressed his palm to my back. He steered me to the bathroom this way without drawing attention.

When we were kids, I used to wrestle with Mykol for fun, rubbing our elbows and knees raw on my parents' orange shag carpet. Because I was older than him, I tended to win, and because I was older, I celebrated my win with the nastiness only brothers practice. Sometimes when I had his shoulders pinned to the ground, I would loom over his face and threaten to drool, sometimes letting a bit start at the corner of my mouth. Our other brother, Rory, would shout, "Do it! Do it! Drool him! Give him a drooling!" I don't think I ever did, but I can't be sure. Now, as Mykol guided me and my pants to the can, I felt rotten for everything I'd ever done to him.

Nobody else was in the washroom. Mykol asked what the problem was, so I extended the waist of my pants to demonstrate.

"And what's wrong with that?" he said. "Looks comfortable."

"Seriously, Mykol, the zipper-waist-control-thing is broken, and I can't tighten them enough to keep them on. Please, can you have a look?"

On my face I mustered a look of innocent encouragement.

"Aw, jeez," he whined as he knelt down, brought his head to my stomach, flipped my waistband over, and began to tug and wrench.

"I don't know what's wrong with it," I began. Two guys

walked into the washroom, spotted us, apologized, and quickly retreated. With the pants to match, I became Jack Tripper in some lost episode.

It didn't take Mykol long to fix my busted zipper. When we left the washroom, I left convinced that I needed to reconsider my eyesight and act a little more carefully with it. I was ashamed, but in a specific sense: mine was the sting that comes with delayed transformation. I felt like a man whose mid-life crisis had caught up, enlightening him to what a bad idea his new earring was, and how silly he looked wearing the same clothes as his son. In that bathroom I left behind something like my youth and, for sure, my few punk rock days. At that specific moment I became worried, cautious, and practical beyond my years, and I was miserable. That was my first feeling for what it meant to be disabled. I felt very old. I had to wear my blindness from now on, whether I found it ill-fitting or not, and I knew it in my bones.

As Mykol and I walked upstairs into the main area of the club, a man descended the steps towards us. By his size and his stride, I knew he was a bouncer. Mykol knew it by the word "Security" on the guy's chest.

When he reached us, he blocked the stairs and asked us to leave the club. Mykol asked why. The bouncer said something to the effect that we knew damn well why and that this wasn't no bathhouse here, man. I didn't want to explain what had happened. Who cares, I thought. It's closing time, anyway.

My brother took a different position. As the bouncer escorted us to the street, Mykol grinned and argued, saying,

"It's just some brotherly love, man! What have you got against brotherly love?"

When I arrived home, the apartment was dark. I didn't bother with the lights. I walked down the hall, feeling my way, and knocked on Jane's door with the heel of my palm. Only lower tones could reach her ears. I heard her wake up, turn in her bed, and tell me to come in. Something became clear in the black of her room, but I can't remember what. I climbed into bed beside her and began to cry. I told Jane everything, how threatened I felt, how scared I was of my eyes, of my future, and of who I was becoming. She stroked my hair and said everything would be okay, everything would look better tomorrow. Her hands undressed me and pulled the blankets over us. We were two tangled and frightened kids, both wounded and hidden away. Our hope was that nothing would find us or take anything more from us. At some point, just before morning, I fell into a deep and colourless sleep. For three years we stayed together that way.

Bodysnatchers from the Planet NASDAQ

Lougheed Highway is ugly and unremarkable. It also feels cold and rough against the back of your head.

I remember waking up, spread-eagled on my back, and staring at a street lamp. Movement felt available to my body, but I didn't feel capable, as they say, of going towards the light. I palmed for my hat and wondered if I'd crushed it in the fall. My time out and away hadn't been long, maybe a few seconds, but that was time enough on the wet asphalt to soak my pants and jacket. My palms, face down on the road, had numbed somewhat, too. That was a sort of booby prize. Shredded skin is best chilled.

Jane and I had taken the bus home from the university that night. We'd gotten off at our usual stop, and stepped into the usual Vancouver rain, ready to hoof the two remaining blocks home. Although the whereabouts of our apartment minimized my noodling around in the dark, our bus stop proved to be an inconvenience. It was on a busy highway, and on return trips from class, we had to cross it. Not one of my great talents.

The highway also challenged my penchant for laziness. The crosswalks in either direction seemed too far, especially in the rain, and especially at night. My eyes detected so little in the dark that walking itself had become a dangerous mode of transportation. Better to shorten the journey by sprinting across the highway, and home. You know you've still got some running left in you, my mind would taunt, although the rest of me would doubt it.

Test run the feeling for yourself some time. In an empty parking lot or an empty ball diamond, close your eyes and sprint a good distance. You'll experience just how unhappy the act makes your body feel. Even when your mind knows it's safe, the rest of you will drag and resist like a mighty skeptic. That inner argument produces a strange, herky-jerky motion, too. Running blind is never pretty, let me tell you, nor smart.

This time, however, my mind didn't prod me to bolt. Jane did. We got off the bus, and she glanced at the pause in traffic and said, "Quick, quick." She was off, so I ran after her with particular abandon. The four lanes were clear for now, but Jane failed to mention the median that interrupted the otherwise level street. I suppose, in all fairness, she didn't know she'd failed to mention anything. Neither of us was too clear about what needed mentioning to me and when. Because my blindness could worsen daily, its effects always seemed somewhat new and unpredictable.

As I ran, I discovered the cement median for myself, with my foot. I tripped, skidded on my hands, rolled, then landed on my back in a lane of oncoming traffic. Jane raced back to fetch me and to stop the approaching cars.

When I came to, she helped me up, dusted me off, and put

my hat back on top of my head, as a mother might do for a toddler after a failed first crack at walking. The rest of the way home I limped and kept my hand fixed to Jane's elbow for guidance. My frustration followed us. I'd just tripped over another of my incompatibilities with life's basic skills. As we walked, and the pain announced itself in my palms and head, Jane asked, carefully, circuitously, if I thought maybe—just maybe—it was time to look into a white cane. For two years I'd avoided the thought, despite twenty-four months of bumping and bruising myself. The tumble, although not the worst I'd taken, amplified my sense of endangerment. I felt stumped for an argument against the inevitable. Pride wasn't enough to refuse a cane. A promise to walk slowly or to even stay home wasn't enough, either. Not anymore. I'd exhausted my own ridiculous solutions. Although I had only been knocked down and out for a few seconds, sometimes that's all it takes. A new world order can emerge when nobody's looking, and fast.

Taking up a white cane is perhaps the most dispiriting thing a newly blinded person goes through. Our mobility aid is a form of confession and defeat. Its battered white segments and red stripe declare the very identity we've always feared, avoided, or hoped to disown. A cane is a permanent commitment to blindness, more final than a diagnosis, even. In my case, I committed to it because, while languishing on Lougheed Highway, I understood, at a molecular level, that I had to adapt to the pressures of an unseen world. If I didn't, I would soon be feeling a lot of other pressures, such as a Honda against my face. I could survive, as long as I could adapt. A white cane substitutes for slow evolution. A cane, albeit primitive and clumsy, also relieves us of one dangerous paradox: the blind are most vulnerable when we are not seen. The entire human species has been through this problem, not that long ago.

About 543 million years back, our gooey, shapeless forebears sprouted the first complex eyes. Seeing had to start somewhere, sometime. According to the biologist Andrew Parker, in his book *In the Blink of an Eye,* the first complex eye to appear on the planet may have evolved in less than a five-hundred-thousand-year period. In terms of evolutionary time, that's no time at all. Imagine if I'd grown, while cuddling the pavement on Lougheed Highway, an eyeball on each earlobe. Profound adaptations can happen in haste. In the blink of an eye, even a white cane can fuse itself to your hand.

Seeing, not to understate the point, transformed the world. For one thing, when the first "eyes" appeared, the oceans of protein blobs and cells and whatnot had to adapt to a new survival pressure. For the first time in history, they were the objects of sight. They were seen but not necessarily able to stare back. Most of the seeing was done by predators who, with this new sense, enjoyed a super-Darwinian advantage. Prey had some major evolving of their own to do, pronto. Developing meaningful and defensive shapes and colours was a start. Another way to put it is this: when sight began in the world, so did the visual meaning of form. To that end, prey might quickly evolve spiky skeletons so predators wouldn't want to take a bite, or prey might suggest toxicity with bright colours. According to Parker's theory, even those that didn't evolve an eye had to adapt to being seen. Sight was inescapable, whether you had it or not. Parker calls this the "Light Switch Theory." The degrees, varieties, and speed of evolutionary change in that period remain unparalleled.

I like to think I've had a taste of it, too. On Lougheed Highway, my own light-switch era began. I had to evolve to meet the pressures of a sighted world, and a cane was, and still is, the best adaptation my body knows. Strictly speaking, it's not evolution, but a cane is as close to sight as technology gets. Like the world 543 million years ago, my switch was also about being seen, not just making up for blindness. If others couldn't see me not seeing them, I needed whatever competitive edge technology could offer. Some call my cane, that extraordinary innovation, by its more common name: stick. We've shuttled greetings beyond our solar system, decoded the human genome, and harvested frozen methane. I have a stick.

Within a week I contacted the Canadian National Institute for the Blind, outed my difficulties, and made an appointment with a mobility instructor. I would be given a white cane and taught how to use it. Funny to think that a person needs to be schooled in the ways of banging a stick, but it's true. There's an art to it. Nobody said it's a dedicated or varied art, but a little technique is involved. How much, I couldn't say at the time.

I'd never been to a CNIB office in all my years on the planet. I'd pretty much steered clear of them and any help they might offer. Now I was on their doorstep and in real need. At the time, mobility training took place in the cellar of a large brown building, one that looked more like military barracks than a nonprofit haven for the squinty. Somehow the building's look reassured me, though, and made me believe this was both an essential and courageous step. This was war, and this was my side's bunker. This was about survival of the fittest in a sighted world, and, dammit, I needed some gadgetry and technique before natural selection sent me the way of the dodo.

Inside the bunker, I waited in the lobby for my instructor. Today, for my first lesson, he'd scheduled some one-on-one training.

I'd read and heard about the intensive instruction people received with guide dogs. For me, a dog was out of the question. It's one thing to commit to a stick, and another to cling to a muddy sidekick named Wally. A dog even eliminates one liberty. To a degree, you can hide blindness, selectively show and conceal your white cane, but you can't hide a golden retriever. As well, I recognized I was still too selfish and immature to be responsible for another living being. The guilt didn't appeal. I would regret sitting at a desk and writing or reading for hours on end while my guide dog sat bored at my feet, secretly hating me and my educational goals or sitcom fetish. Then there was the matter of my permanent disinterest in Frisbee. A dog was out of the question.

I only hoped that my training with a stick would differ greatly from the kind of training given with guide dogs. What I'd read and heard suggested mobility instructors liked to place a blind person and her new dog in perilous situations—

walking along edges, or into traffic, or through minefields, that sort of thing. That didn't appeal. Dropping me off, say, at night, in an unknown neighbourhood and telling me to find my way home with only a length of white fiberglass with a golf club handle for assistance—well, if that was my training, I'd rather stay home forever. Maybe just a little training, just the basics, would be enough.

I stood waiting in the lobby for a few minutes. Soon a wiry man in heavy glasses burst from behind a door. He came at me with his open hand, as a mugger might with a fishing knife. This was a man whose hand needed shaking, and bad. So much, in fact, that he snatched mine from my side before I could offer it. Only later would it occur to me that he couldn't be sure I'd seen his greeting, so he took responsibility for the ritual. That memory is my clearest of the day. It may be the first time somebody ever approached me as a blind person.

"Hi," he said. "Ryan, right? I'm Jimmy. I'll be your m-m-mobility instructor today."

We'd spoken briefly on the phone, and I recognized his voice. The stutter, too.

"Today?" I asked. "Will this take more than today?"

"Just a few—a few—" His stutter hamstrung him on the next word, so he changed the approach. "It won't take long," he said.

He placed my hand on his elbow for guidance. Together we made our way through several corridors. The place seemed to be bursting at the edges. Boxes and broken chairs and the odd table crowded the hallways, stuff pushed and stacked to the sides. Maybe these obstacles would be part of my training, I thought. I paid attention and memorized what I could. If training wouldn't take long, I'd make it take even less time.

Our final turn brought us into a stairwell that we descended, until we emerged into the bowels of the bunker. A large, open, and musty concrete basement. A few orange pylons peppered the floor, and a few large support beams interrupted the open training space. Otherwise, two men were off in a corner, one of them rhythmically tapping a cane while the other offered praise. The room was dim. I could hardly make out a thing. I only heard the two men, and I only knew of the pillars and pylons because Jimmy yanked me around them, saying, "Watch out for the pylon on your left," or "We're passing a post on your right." Extra letters accompanied his descriptions. I don't mean to mock them, either. The stutter remains something memorable and good. I felt more at ease because of it. We were both somewhat vulnerable and, in our own ways, hesitant.

From a rack of canes on the wall, Jimmy selected a few, measured them, and chose one that stood chest-high. He showed me how to collapse the stick into its four short segments and how the cane could be quickly reassembled with a flick of the handle, allowing the lengths to drop and the elastic cord to naturally pull the cane back into shape.

"Quick to store, quick to retrieve," he noted. High-speed camouflage, I thought.

Next we used one of the pillars. My first lesson would be about swinging the cane for maximum defence. The cane, Jimmy explained, is held at a forty-five-degree angle to the ground, lifted, and swung left and right. The outside edges are tapped. Don't drag or wipe. Lift and swing.

"When I step forward with my left foot," he said, "I should be t-tapping on the right. This way I know nothing is where my right foot will g-g-go."

Made sense to me. I tried the method out and became a walking metronome. Caning is a perpetual rhythm. You do, quite literally, walk to the beat of your own drum. A beat also involves beating on something. That was our next concern. Jimmy aligned me a good distance from a pillar and tasked me with some deliberate stick work.

"Now, I want you to cl-cl-close your eyes, no cheating with what you've got, and walk towards the post. Use your cane and st-st-stop when you tap the obstacle in front of you."

I did as I was told, closed my eyes—not that I could see much, anyway—and walked directly towards the pillar. After a couple of steps, a more natural rhythm with the cane emerged, but I slowed. I knew something was coming. I could feel it, but not with the cane, not yet. My anticipation swung out further. It felt for what I knew must be inevitable. After a few more steps, I still hadn't connected, so I slowed down even more, breaking into a pronounced stutter-step. I worried my cane would miss the pillar, and that worry lit in me a familiar but curious sensation. Vertigo. Walking in the dark, unsure of what's to come, is closest in feeling to walking off the edge of a cliff. Each step was into nothing until I felt firm and empty ground under my foot again. The edge of the world is always the next step when you're blind.

Then Jimmy spoke with what sounded like urgency.

"S-s-s—" he began, so I stopped. Maybe I was about to clip the pillar or trip over a pylon or— "S-super! Keep it straight," he said, "you're doing great! Maybe pick up the pace a bit. You'll learn to t-trust the cane after a while."

I resumed my shuffle. Soon enough, my cane whacked the pillar. Artificial sight rattled through my hand and up my arm. From now on, that would be my way of looking. Not a subtle vibration of light but clunky, whopping frictions in my muscles. I was groping and pawing about the face of the planet, like my ancient forebears. I was primal.

"Good," Jimmy said, "now follow my voice and we'll try the stairs."

At the foot of the staircase he took my cane and showed me how to tap the lip of the steps as I ascended them. The sound carried a memory. I was a kid again, running a stick along a neighbour's fence. Or maybe that was a movie about a kid and a fence. Either way, the technique transformed a little boy's pleasure into a set of eyes. When the sound stops, Jimmy explained, when there's nothing left to tap, you know the next step is the final one. Then he showed me how to descend. Hold the cane parallel with the decline of the stairs, he said, and let the tip extend below. The cane connects with the ground first and tells you when the stairs finish. Again, it all made sense. Such a simple and elegant solution for the complex eye. I tried it out, and it worked. We had stairs, and we had obstacles down tight. Now it was time for the building ledges and open sewer covers.

"G-g-great," Jimmy said. "Any questions?"

"Nope. Seems clear enough. What's next?"

"That's it. You're r-ready. Call if you have any questions."

"That's it?" I couldn't imagine every situation solved with just those two techniques. "What about, I don't know, traffic?"

Jimmy laughed. "If you can touch it with your cane, you're too c-c-close."

My training, in the end, took as much time from my life as morning toast. My new complex eye wasn't that complex after all. When I stepped outside, I tried my caning technique on the sidewalk. Then, feeling ridiculous for swinging it across what I knew was a clear and open path, I stuffed my stick in my backpack and caught a bus home. My cane stayed in the bag for several weeks. I had an aid, but despite its handiness, I had yet to truly take it on. That would be the next evolutionary stage, if I could make it.

The problem was this. Only after accidents or near-accidents would I think, shit, you know, I really should take that thing out of my crud bag. Maybe I'd think that after bouncing my nose off a vending machine or sitting on the lap of what I took to be an empty chair. After moments like these, I'd flirt with the idea of my cane or haul the actual stick out for a little while. But when I grew safe and confident again, back into my bag it went. I treated my mobility aid like I treated my blindness: both were occasional. Keeping them camouflaged was a temptation I couldn't resist, as long as I wasn't being outed by an accident. To really commit to the cane, something more had to give. Because I didn't always need it, I had to go one step beyond. I had to want it.

Wanting to cane is a challenge, counterintuitive as it may

sound. I may not need a cane at every waking moment, but that doesn't mean I can put it down until I say, hey, here comes another pesky phone booth, better get out the trusty old stick. Although we may be blind all the time, that doesn't mean we're always uncertain about what is around us. To keep my cane in hand I had to learn to enjoy its certainty and potential, even when neither seemed necessary. That's a difficult lesson.

Put it this way. If nobody's around, and everything is safe, how does somebody enjoy a stick? Even more difficult, how is a stick enjoyed when everybody else is watching? I think of that poor Star Wars Kid on the Internet. One day, at school, he videotaped himself playing Jedi knight. Bad idea. He made the sound effects with his lips, swung a broom handle like a light saber, and danced and battled as only a Jedi can. Then somebody outed him. Some doofus classmate came along, found the tape and, having eaten too much paste in elementary school, proceeded to upload the footage to the web. The cult following that ensued, and its mockery of the Star Wars Kid, are global.

I think I can identify, even though the scale is different. I mean, if this poor kid was the Death Star of embarrassing situations, proportionately speaking, I was the freight elevator on Level 12. I, too, felt for weeks that whenever I swung my own stick, everybody in the world caught a glimpse of me. I was playing Blind Man for the crowd. Hey, look at me! I'm acting like a guy who needs a stick. Even I don't think I need one right now, so I'll casually swing it around until it seems useful again. In effect, I'd grown so accustomed to the secrecy, the privacy, of my condition, that I wasn't prepared to be seen yet.

Denying my blindness wasn't my own job, either. Not anymore. Many faces joined in on the work. Within my shrinking tunnel vision, I glimpsed people's expressions of confusion, derision, suspicion, and surprise as I tapped past. In these faces I found too much accusation. I didn't look blind to them or blind enough, not all the time, and I still don't on occasion. What could I do, though? Stop and describe my pathology after every sidelong look? For the first few weeks, the shame was powerful enough to keep my cane in my backpack.

Eventually I nursed a small shift in perspective. Somehow I stopped looking at myself just long enough to discover the terrific and strange power I had over others. With a cane I could conjure dynamics just too wicked to put down. The awkwardness I caused some sighted people made the cane easier to hang on to while I grew accustomed to its use. I caused chaos. That was my methadone, my Nicorette gum, and my crutch. It was the cane for my cane. Here's an example.

Typical reactions to a white cane separate sighted people into several distinct groups. The most common behaviour is exhibited by a group I'll call the Stumps. They are people who, despite a wide walkway, be it a parking lot or mall or even a Canadian prairie, see a blind person approaching, perhaps a hundred yards away or a hundred feet, and then quietly wait. Instead of stepping aside or indicating their presence with some noise—a grunt, a shriek of terror, a "Look out, I'm just ahead of you"—instead of a simple coping technique, Stumps fix in place. They are stumped. They hope that somehow the blind person heading their way will

magically change course. Stumps seem to survive and perpet-
uate their useless activity only because the blind have not yet
evolved enough weight or speed, like a car, to make our
impact enough to wipe out the Stumps one at a time. Of
course some of them feel regret. Some apologize, too, and are
sincerely sorry for not moving. The apologists are Stumps
who've added a moral dimension to their paralysis. They're
kind but draining. Everybody feels rotten for everybody else.

My favourite people are still the Jiggers. Given a wide berth
and a long, plain view of an approaching white cane, Jiggers
paralyse, then boogie at the last second. They threaten to bolt
left, then right, then left again, indecisive and panic-stricken,
until either a direction is chosen or, more times then not, they
dance in place until impact. Their dance is best described as
the same one managed by all grade eight boys who can't
dance. You know the moves. Their arms lock at a ninety-
degree angle and swing, their fists chug up and down, and
their hips sway with self-consciousness, all this to the rhythm
of their own bouncity-bounce. Totally neat. Unfortunately, I
think they do it in front of cars, too, so I meet fewer of these
folks.

Everybody else is great. They hear and see you coming,
and they go like creek water around a rock. The groups above
were helpful, though. They're an example of what made a
cane just too strange a thing to put down. It's too fun to cause
that much trouble, too intoxicating to upset the expectations
of daily, public routine. A white cane causes as much slapstick
as it prevents. Whenever I felt awkward in public, I saw I
wasn't alone. I wasn't the only one who had mobility issues.

My perspective changed in other, more serious, and material ways. For one thing, the world shrank. Walking along a city street, inside my own darkness, my cane keeps me focused on these few intimate points of here and now, on this little patch I swipe at. Each tap of my cane is comparable to opening an eye, a brief glance, then my eye lifts and swings, closing again, until it taps the other side, winking at this and that. My sense of the view became tactile, not colourful; immediate, not distant. Something within arm's reach.

The cane also changed my disposition. Because it concentrates me on the "here" and the "now," I probably won't die of hypertension. Mine is a relaxing passage through space. A cane keeps the focus on what is present and in front of me. I am never in a hurry, because I don't think of "there," only "here." I'm interested in my next step, and I make it carefully. My pace is slow, not resentful of having a long way to go or too impatient, say, to use a crosswalk. What I tap is where I am and what I'm doing. It's nice living in the here and now. My cane made me this way, and I can't say with certainty I'd be of the same spirit without it.

The downside of caning is that, like the prey of so many millions of years ago, I'm different because I'm seen now: people recognize me as a blind man and act accordingly. I'm conspicuous, like a minor celebrity, even. I'm the blind guy around here. That can create a false sense of safety. In some respects I take less care when walking around, less caution than I did in my caneless incarnation. Before, I used to worry about both not seeing something and not being recognized as a blind man. If I walked through a crowded mall, I had to try and move around people because I couldn't assume they'd notice me, and I couldn't assume that they would steer clear of this guy who happens to be shuffling in a funny way. Now that I have a cane, I tend to assume people see me, and they do. That's why I take more risks. Not huge ones, but risks all the same. When I step into traffic because I think it's safe, I trust my cane will stop everything. Usually it does. I hope never to be proven wrong.

Without question, my stick is a part of my past and present life. But it certainly isn't the future. Soon I may have other gadgetry, new technologies that will, one day, replace this cane and fuse me with some new digital resolve. A person with a white cane is an emerging cyborg. A stick is a primitive beginning, but soon enough my flesh and machinery will merge into a new being. That's the next step of my evolution, and it may happen in my lifetime.

Among other places, I often wonder if my future is in Naperville, Illinois. There, two brothers, doctors Vincent and Alan Chow, are developing the first artificial retina. A microchip retina. The device is less than two millimetres in diameter and not quite as thick as a human hair. The artificial retina contains roughly five thousand photosensitive cells that generate an electrical signal when exposed to light. No batteries or extension cords are needed. When implanted, this extra retina would artificially stimulate my natural retina cells, jump-starting them into action again. The theory is predicated on the fact that seeing happens in the brain, not the eye. Signals are all the eye creates, and those signals are interpreted by the brain into images. I've still got a brain, I think.

I just need a new interface with the code of light. One day, maybe. For now, the stick remains my best and only prosthetic, although others, like the microchip retina, are busy fashioning what I may one day become.

I say all of that with caution. My generation never had a Woodstock, not really. But Silicon Valley, before the NASDAQ bubble burst in the late 1990s, may have been the closest my generation has come to our own utopian-flavoured lost weekend. I keep it in mind as a cautionary tale about my possible cure and imminent rebirth as a cyborg. So many shiny objects are out there in the technological playground, and we all know how much the sighted like shiny objects. Sometimes we make magnificent things out of them. Canes, for example. Yet, sometimes shininess is all our fantasies are about. I don't know if I could ever commit myself to implanting a piece of technology in my body, knowing one day it will necessarily follow the eight-track tape, the abacus, and Pong. My cane works well, but would I surgically attach it to my arm? Technologies, like species, adapt and disappear at their own extraordinary pace, too. I find it hard to imagine what it would take for me to commit to a technology other than my cane. A solid performance on NASDAQ probably won't be enough.

For now, I try to remember what my eyes have shown me. The more complex something is, the more difficult, when broken, it is to cope. Everything breaks. Better a stick than an eye, or a stick than a microchip. With something like a cane, at least my independence extends to fixing the problem. Something small as a stick can change your whole being. The fantasy grows from there, and so do I.

I remember when my mother and I stood outside the doctor's office one afternoon. I'd recently picked up my cane and graduated from the mobility training. She hadn't seen me use the stick yet, and the image of it frightened her. Until that moment, my blindness, for her, was relatively abstract. Blindness was a diagnosis about the future, a disease with a name, and some clumsiness in my manner. But now I had a cane, and the sight of it proved my condition. We stood on the corner, outside the office building, and waited for the crosswalk signal to change. Ma tapped the sidewalk with my cane, testing its version of the world. The sound and the image were both frightening to me, too. My mother with a white cane. Now I knew something about how I must have looked to her.

"Is this how you're supposed to do it?" she asked, and dragged the cane across the concrete, precisely as Jimmy had discouraged.

"Not exactly," I said.

"Here, you show me how it works."

Ma handed me my cane. As a nearby bus pulled away, I edged to the street and swung the stick, clipping the side of the bus as it passed.

"Hear that?" I said. "Sounds grey."

Ma laughed. "Very fancy. A cane that tells colour."

Whatcha Got

The New Orleans I remember, the one before the floods, loved a good hustle. Don't get me wrong, I say this with respect and gratitude. I too love a good sleight-of-hand. The New Orleans I remember offered plenty. The last days of Jane and Ryan fit in well there. We'd fooled ourselves as long as we could, until there was no going home. Sometimes we build on hope, shaky as it is. Sometimes it isn't enough.

My relationship with her had substantially thinned over three years. To be fair, I don't think she considered me such a peachy catch by the end, either. Rightly so. Time and time again we discovered we had shrinking little in common. On any given Saturday night Jane made crafts at the kitchen table, while I continued to bar-hop with my old friends. A quick nose around the apartment suggested some of our differences, too. You'd find Jane's water-logged Victorian novels neatly stacked beside the bathtub, and maybe a couple of scented candles burning in the corner. My stuff sprawled everywhere else. Piles of my dippy avant-garde poetry covered the living room floor. So did my empty cigarette packs and cassette tapes. Jane perpetually tidied my mess, and I perpetually suffered her lack of hearing aids. Typically they remained on the kitchen table instead of in her ears.

Conversation was always hard, but it atrophied over time. Still, I knew I could communicate in other ways. If I had to hear Enya one more time, I could always throw Jane's Birkenstocks out the window. Frequently I stayed up late listening to the TV or drinking beer and brooding, while Jane went off to bed by herself. I may have been a little blinder than before, but things didn't look good.

Our demise wasn't dramatic or attached to a specific moment, really. Like my vision, we went out in a slow blur. Disability first brought us together, but eventually it dissolved our affections, too. I didn't want to talk about my eyes much, not with Jane, not with anybody, even though my tunnel vision continued to decay and horrify. I thought I was coping, but I could only laugh off so much. Not the bitterness and anger. With nothing tangible to rage against, soon I targeted our relationship. Over time, our mutual acceptance and comfort soured into resentment. In Jane I stopped seeing anything but my frailty, my need for safety and my fear of loneliness. That's all I saw, and that self-loathing grew enough to eclipse the Jane I once knew.

For three years we hid out together, nevertheless. The idea of our early comfort and ease was hard to give up, especially because we didn't know what we'd be giving it up for. Who could desire a blind man or a deaf woman? A break-up could be for nothing, and that's why we tried to mend our imminent split. A vacation, we thought, a vacation might do us some good.

During our last summer, we packed up Jane's hearing aids and my white cane and went through the considerable frustration of navigating our bodies, as uncooperative as ever, from Vancouver to Louisiana. It wasn't intended solely to be a couple's retreat. We travelled for the standard reasons, as well. We went for the jazz, the history, the architecture, the food, and, by all means, those alligator smiles. Who can resist the elegance of a finely honed con game? Not me.

Consider the central scene. In the French Quarter, on Bourbon Street and its neighbouring boulevards, dozens of enterprising kids were at work. They artfully pried change from the fingers of tourists, all of it well deserved. The first hook I heard went something like this.

"Hey, mister," a kid said, "c'mon mister, you got two bucks? Betcha two bucks I can tell you where you got your shoes."

I knew it was a sucker's game, but that's what I was buying, even seeking. I wanted to lose, to be the good loser, as did all the other tourists who swallowed his hook. I was tickled to be deceived, as in a magic show or the land of Oz. The pleasure, in the end, was in discovering what I couldn't see, even if it was merely a pun lurking somewhere in the question. The lift of revelation only cost two bucks, to boot. That's cheaper than microchip retinas, snake handling, psychoanalysis, or any other means to revelation I can think of.

"Okay, I'm in," I said, caning my way back towards the voice I had just passed.

It was late afternoon, and I'd given up on Jane by this point. She was still off somewhere in a shop looking at bric-a-brac. All day she'd been at it, and she didn't seem to have a plan to quit. Now was my chance to take in some of the

colourful repertoire around me. My version of sight-seeing.
I like taking in fresh language uses of any kind.

"Here's your two bucks. Okay, tell me where I got my
shoes."

I waited for an answer, but all I received was an awkward
silence. Then the kid began to fill it in with some stammering.

"Uh, well, uh," he said, "Like, I, actually, I was talking to
this guy here."

Great, I thought, now I look like a street arts zealot. How
often does someone burst in as if he can't live another second
without learning where he got his shoes? By the measure of
our pause, I'd say my zealotry was, in fact, rare. The kid
quickly recovered his patter and rhythm, the lifeblood of his
hustle.

"But, hey," he began, "ain't nothing wrong with your
money. It's at least as good as this guy's, eh? Four bucks it is,
and I'll tell everybody here where everybody got their shoes,
all four of 'em. Unless one of you got some third leg tucked
away somewheres. You know—*kickstanding*."

I'm going to guess the kid leaned to demonstrate whatever
kickstanding looked like. I'm not sure. Nobody laughed,
either way.

"On second thought," the man said, the one I'd barged in
on, "I think I've changed my mind. That's okay, you go ahead
with this guy."

"No way! No need, no need," the kid said, "I got plenty for
everybody. You watch, you just watch me. I can, you know—
multi-task. Mul-ti-task!"

"I dunno," the man said, "maybe I should—hey, I may not even have the two dollars, come to think of it."

The man stood just outside my tunnel vision. The sound of loose change jingled as he rummaged through his pockets. Under his breath, he debated spending the money, deeply uncertain, as if about to buy a black market kidney.

"C'mon, mister," the kid cut in, "It's just two bucks. There's plenty of shoes for everybody. Just gimme what you got there, and that's good enough. We'll be, like, *square*."

I liked the way this kid pumped something else out of words, although I don't know exactly what. Apparently square and multitask don't mean *square* and *multitask*. Finally the man next to me arrived at a decision.

"You know what? I think I'm gonna say no. I think I've changed my mind. You go ahead and tell this guy where he got his shoes and I'll keep my shopping habits to myself." He chuckled at his own turn of phrase. "Heh, heh, heh. I'm happy to just watch, thanks."

But the kid and I both knew Scrooge McTourist wanted a free kick. You know his kind. He was one of those misers who'll stop to listen to a busker, then either pretend to drop something in the hat or, if the hat is passed, pretend hats don't really exist.

"Here," I said, "here's four bucks. Give us the works."

"No! No, please don't." Scrooge was upset. "You don't have to pay for me. I'm fine. Save your money. I'll just watch."

There's nothing like the poor blind man paying for the stingy tourist. I enjoyed that I could boost his free ride and enjoyed that he couldn't do anything about it. Hostage takings are nice.

"No, I insist," I said. "Here, four bucks."

I held my fist out in front of me. From it dangled four bills. Nobody took them. It seemed Scrooge and the kid didn't know how to handle my gesture.

Reluctance like theirs is common, and it interests me. For many, when a blind person tries to pay, something awkward happens. Even with everything on the up and up in a normal, dull shopping moment, my cash becomes jinxed or toxic or something. It's a funny social impropriety, what my money and I can cause. In some people, I sense a moral complication happens. They act tentative with me, as if taking a blind man's money is an abuse. It's really fun. But I suspect the situation is something more dynamic. Their caution isn't so much a reaction to my blindness or my filthy blind man's money, Rather, cashiers and sales clerks are caught off guard by my body language and its unintended meaning. I don't hand the cash over, I hold it out to be taken. That's an upsetting shift, for some, having to take instead of receive. Especially from the gimpy.

I felt uncomfortable, too, waiting like that, my hand in the air, posed like one of those obnoxious cigar store Indians. I suppose I could've tossed the bills down into the kid's hat but that might have seemed insulting. Who said there was a hat, anyway? The bills might have fluttered to the hatless sidewalk, as if to say, "Here you go, here's your stinking money. Now pick it up!" I've learned not to toss anything. Too dangerous. Once, in Berlin, I was eating cherries as I strolled my friend's neighbourhood. Breezing along, I tried to spit a pit into a public garbage can, but what I took to be a trash bin turned out to be an elderly and surprised fräulein on a bench. To this day I launch nothing in any direction.

"Here," I instructed, and waggled the money some more. "Just take it and tell us where we got our shoes."

The three of us had successfully killed any fun any joke could deliver. The kid finally tugged the four bills from my hand, as gentle as could be.

"You got your shoes on your feet, fools."

An extra dollar remained between my fingers. I'd taken five from my wallet by accident.

The kid and I joked around a bit, then chatted a while about business in the Quarter, about our homes, about his other gags, about my blindness. Eventually, before I left, with Scrooge McTourist long gone, the kid took my hand, shook it, and palmed me two bucks back.

"No, you keep it," I said, but he insisted I take the two bills.

It hadn't occurred to me that we'd become partners. If I didn't take the money, there'd be no punch line. If I took the money back, we'd conned the stingy guy together. He'd always think the poor blind man paid his way when the poor blind man hadn't shelled out anything. I thanked the kid for a good time and pocketed our winnings.

My vacation wasn't all about that kind of con, though. It goes without saying I wouldn't have gone through the fresh hell of travelling a different country and a new city with my white cane, not just for bad jokes. Leaving my routine and my

neighbourhood kicks out the crutch of memory. In that
respect, my home is perhaps the only spot on the planet
where I can truly feel secured within a rich sense of place.
Always will be.

When I say home, I mean two things. More than the apartment I live in today, I'm thinking of the places I walk to in my
neighbourhood and everything I've memorized within that
distance.

My mental map is not to be underestimated. I've memorized this neighbourhood in excruciating and ridiculous
detail, a degree the sighted would pay no mind. Rarely will
you find me venturing beyond that knowledge and the places
it circumscribes. Where I live is a state of mind, quite literally.
It's a matter of defence, even delusion. Memory keeps me
from being as thoroughly blind as I am. When you can't see,
nothing seems to exist in a city or landscape if it isn't in mind
already.

Think about buildings. Each one I passed in Louisiana
appeared to be, and remained, a vague sketch of an idea, no
more and no less. I saw bits of its shape, and that's all. An
unknown like that repels me because it's too overwhelming,
with all its capacity to hurt, embarrass, disorient, and elude.
Sighted people walking past new places ask, "What's in
there?" The blind ask, "What's that?" We are far, far away,
even when we are near.

When I do muster the courage and wherewithal to venture
inside the shape of an unknown building, I can, with a lot of
effort, error, and discomfort, touch my way into some limited
knowledge of the contents and purposes served there. Only

then, in a sense, have I seen what most people glean as they walk by, or derive from reading the store sign. If I can't touch something, if it isn't narrated to me, it isn't there. So I pay no mind to what I don't know. I only go where I remember.

As you might imagine, disorientation takes on a whole new meaning. When I travel, the scale of being lost is different than when I was sighted. It's not about directions, not at the street level anymore, although that's always a problem. More immediate is the sense that, say, sitting in a new bar in a new city, when I let go of my beer, along with it I let go of the surety it imparts about where I am and what's around me. I can easily feel I'm nowhere. The sensation compounds and follows me, too. The world away from home doesn't make my world bigger. It introduces me to a terrifying smallness. It's like moving from living in a complex city map to a skeletal line drawing.

Back home, the bus stop is twenty paces from the corner of Fifth Avenue. No bench. The stop is beside a tree, and I know where to wait because of the branches that graze my porkpie hat. The bank machine nearest my house is around the corner and inside the first set of doors. Only the right one opens. I don't read the screens on the ATM. I don't have to. I've memorized the pattern of buttons to press and in what order to press them. At Slickity Jim's Chat and Chew, Tyler always puts the cream for my coffee beside the mug's handle and puts the sugar beside my napkin. The others who work there tell me at what time they've placed my sandwich, quick and habitual. The washroom is to the left of the open kitchen door. These memories make the basics of my lunch hour map at home. I haven't even mentioned how I know which key is which on my ring, how I've memorized the menus of several restaurants, according to my tastes, how I've memorized grocery store aisles, how I've learned which intersections could trick me into crossing when cars are turning left in front of me, and so on and so on.

But here, in New Orleans, or anywhere else in the world, where do they keep the cream? Which of these buildings could be a bank? Which door is for the bank machine and which buttons do I press in what order? How do I know from out here on the sidewalk that this bank isn't a mattress store? Every gesture, step, reach for the cream, when I'm away from home, is a grope and test to see if anything is in front of me, let alone the particular thing I'm looking for. I'm always on the edge, then, of a flat and shrunken earth, trying my best to give it more dimension. That's closer to exploring than holidaying or travelling, and we all know how rested explorers feel.

So, why go to New Orleans, then, or anywhere? My only answer is this: self-delusion. I always think travelling this time will be different. I always hope it will get better. Every time. Maybe I could be conned into having a different experience— that's my hope. That was my hope in New Orleans and my hope for my relationship with Jane, too.

The first morning of our trip, we left the hostel and cut our way across the small patch of lawn beside the entrance. We debated breakfast as we left. Jane wanted beignets at Café du Monde, and I wanted catfish as fast as humanly possible, especially if we could get it at Igor's Bar, Grill, and

Laundromat. I mostly wanted to see who the hell would be in a bar, grill, and laundromat at seven o'clock in the morning.

Not two or three steps across the lawn, Jane let out a screech and bolted for the sidewalk, her knees lifting as she ran. In her blurry shape I remembered images I'd seen in high school biology class, some bit of film footage of a Jesus lizard getting up the speed to run on water. I, on the other hand, froze in my tracks and awaited further instruction.

It's a funny difference in blindness. If I'm alarmed, my flight-or-fight instinct short-circuits. I can't run, of course, not without jacking up the amount of danger I'd be in. But I can't fight, either, because, well, fight what, where, and how? So, when alarmed, I paralyse in position, then wait, like the passenger I am, for instructions. My method doesn't work very well. Sometimes I have to remind people that I'm still in a holding pattern. This time, Jane, too busy screaming, had forgotten me.

"What! What what what?" I said. I was glued to my spot and unsuccessfully scanning about for clues. "You gotta tell me what's going on!" Snakes, I worried, if it's my luck, it'll be a snake. Jane's sprint had taken her to the sidewalk, where she seemed to feel safe. Safe from whatever I was hanging out with.

"What, what, what?" I reminded her.

"Bugs! Around you on the ground. Really big!"

I looked down at my feet but don't know why. I couldn't see anything, not even in the clean tunnel of my good eye. All I could make out was a blended spectrum of green and brown and yellow. Grass? Grass laced with brown bugs? Brown grass with yellow bugs? Which is worse? Nothing seemed to be moving.

"Hey, guess what?" I said, bringing my face closer to the dirt. "I don't see them."

A man exited the hostel and walked past me along the walkway, the proper path to the sidewalk.

"They're cicada shells," he said. "They look just like live ones, but they're molted shells."

"Could have fooled me," I said.

I gave into beignets for breakfast to help calm Jane's startled heart. In return, we ate dinner that night around the corner at Igor's and closed the day there, courting deception one last time.

I wanted to stay out late and long into the night. We were in New Orleans, after all, and the people we'd met at Igor's were travelling to Vancouver, of all places. Conversation is something I can have and enjoy. Blindness doesn't matter. But Jane's body and character didn't share my sociability or pleasure in a long sit and a long yabber with strangers. Although we helped each other with our disabilities, we didn't always lead one another to a mutual sense of belonging. Jane wanted to go back to the hostel, but I protested we should stay at Igor's. She was bored and wanted to go. Soon, I said, but what she meant was go, as in go now.

Conversations in loud places like Igor's didn't filter well in Jane's hearing aids. The background and the foreground blended, sometimes one taking over from the other. Jane inevitably felt outside the group, not part of the exchange or able to track what was said. I remember how, that night, she would say something, make an observation, and be met by people's confusion. Why does she repeat things we talked about a minute ago? Why does she suddenly talk about chess when we're talking about jazz? Unlike my cane, Jane could hide her hearing aids under her hair, and, often to her detriment, she preferred to keep it that way. Our new bar-buddies didn't know what to make of her. A couple more times her elbow ribbed me, indicating it was time to go, but I pretended not to notice.

True, it was insensitive, but I'd been bored earlier for hours while she looked at knick-knacks. You can only touch so many saxophone lamps or paddleboat snow domes without beating them against your head. I figured, selfishly, it was my turn to do my thing. I wanted to talk with people and sit, two things I can do well. This way we'd be, you know—*square*. The fight was on. A silent one.

I got up to plug some money into the jukebox. No better way to suggest staying. Jane didn't offer to help me, which wasn't our usual routine. Stubborn, I followed the last few bars of the Monkees until I felt the jukebox in front of me, fingered the coin slot, put in my money, and pressed three random selections. I couldn't read the play list, which Jane would normally have helped me with, but anything was better than the Monkees. My first song kicked in. "Daydream Believer."

I found my way back to our table, irritable and ready to stand my ground. Jane got the last word, though, and won the argument. She'd up and left while I was picking songs.

If I was sighted, that would have been fine with me. Our hostel wasn't far from Igor's, just down the street several blocks and a couple of turns, in fact. Then it occurred to me I had no more detail than that in my mental map. I couldn't find the hostel on my own. I knew how Scrooge McTourist must have felt. Jane had hijacked the argument and forced me to go along with her.

I excused myself, left what I guessed to be enough to cover our bill, and chased out the door. Jane waited just outside, certain I'd follow, but I didn't know that. I made it to the corner before she let me know she was right behind. The street was as black as our mood, and I resented the dark as much as I resented my reliance on Jane.

We walked in a silent fury, her stride taking her slightly ahead. Her distance refused me her guiding elbow, but I was happy not to take it. Then a voice from behind me yelled something. Footsteps hustled after me. I stopped and turned to face two large shadows as one of them crowded me and spoke.

"Yo, man. Whatcha got?"

I shrugged. "Huh?"

The other shadow elaborated, very loudly. "He asked you whatcha got, man? Fuckin', whatcha got?"

The two shadows crowded closer. They either had a poor sense of personal space, or they were deliberately jostling me. I couldn't say for sure, but I had a hunch. Then again, people often think I'm deaf because I'm blind. Strangers will press close to my face and holler phrases such as, "You are doing very well at walking!"

"Are you asking what I've got?" I said. "You mean this?" I held up my cane. "It's for the blind."

I'm not entirely stupid. Something felt wrong, even threatening. But asking me "Whatcha got?" was ambiguous at best. I hoped I could answer the question with my cane. The crowding worried me, but I couldn't determine what the intentions of my two shadows were. Facial expressions often complete these pictures.

I'd been mugged once before, but never as a blind man. More accurately, I'd received an amateur thumping from some yahoo when I was fifteen. He, too, started with a cryptic question I couldn't follow.

My friend Chris and I were walking home one night when a gold Camaro zoomed past us, then locked its brakes, and backed up in a hurry. We knew that wasn't good. We hoped it would keep going, but the car parked beside us, in the middle of the street, the engine still running. In a suburb like Langley a gold Camaro is never a good sign, nor is any car that bothers to back up to you and your goth-loving, pointy-toed shoes. You can't run in those things, which was often a problem when I was fifteen.

A long-haired guy in a leather vest and a beer shirt burst from the Camaro and slammed the door. I could hear Iron Maiden on his stereo. Leather vests were another one of Langley's more popular bad signs.

"Where's the fight!?" he shouted, both declaring and asking at the same time. Chris and I couldn't tell what this guy was getting at. "Where's the fight? The fighting-fight?!" he shouted.

I made the mistake of floating an answer. "I dunno?" I said.

Then he showed me where the fight was. Duh, it was here and now. I could smell sour booze breath as he got in my face. He closed in enough to grab me by the head, as if about to pull me in for a nice kiss. But instead of coaxing my lips towards his, like they do in the movies, he slammed my chin into his raised right knee. Several times. Bobbing for kneecaps. A Friday night in Langley.

In New Orleans, when those two shadows asked me what I got, that Camaro memory tore through my body. The crowding reminded me of Mr. Camaro, as did the weird use of a question before a possible drubbing. My answer, I supposed, would begin whatever violence or theft was about to happen.

And why does it have to be so manipulative, anyway? It's like someone asking you, "Hey, do you think the garbage needs to be taken out?" when they really mean to say, "Hey, take the goddamn garbage out." Or, it's like when somebody asks, "What are you going to do about it?" but it really means, in certain circumstances, "Go on and hit me first, please." If my two shadows just outright said, "Give me your money," I would have. But, no, instead we danced with semantics, and I offered them my white cane. In the end, their "Whatcha got?" probably saved me. And the fact Jane was there.

Before they said anything about my cane, or how spiffy it was, or how it wasn't what they were after, I felt Jane's hand snatch my elbow and pull. We walked quickly, and that is a hard thing for a blind person to do with any conviction or grace.

We scooted around the corner a couple of blocks. When Jane couldn't see them anymore, we resumed our usual pace, this time with my hand on her guiding elbow.

"What the hell was that about?" I asked. "I think they wanted my money or something. They asked what I had, and I said this was my cane. But I don't think that's what they were asking."

Before I could say anything more, I heard footsteps coming from behind us, again. Fast footsteps.

My shoulders hunched the way someone might brace themselves against an oncoming dump truck. Jane turned when I froze, saw my shadowmen, and bolted. This time, in her own self-preserving haste, she forgot to take me with her. The two men were on either side of me all over again. They still had issues with personal space.

"Hey, man!" one of them yelled, although they didn't need to get my attention. "You gotta understand somethin', know what I'm saying?"

I nodded, but I hadn't a clue. I figured I would soon enough.

"We, like, didn't know y'all couldn't see nothin', like, bein' blind and all, and so we just wanted to say sorry, know what I'm sayin'?"

"No problem, no worry," I sputtered.

"Yeah," the other voice said, "sorry about that shit. You look like fucking some normal guy, you know what I'm sayin'? You look like just some guy, and we didn't mean to get into your shit or nothin'. You don't look like a blind guy, you know that?"

I nodded in agreement.

"And I respect your peoples and what you got to deal with, man. We cool?"

My people and I were cool. The two men patted me once on the shoulder as they left, as if we were buddies, or I was a pet.

Although I was fine, that night didn't sit well with me for the rest of our trip. Something had, in the end, been taken from me, something very small. A strange kind of dignity, maybe. In its place remained an alien resentment. I know it seems daft, really, but how does one get justice for not having been mugged? It's a real question, although not a high priority. For what it's worth, I learned this much—even commonplace violence and social dangers can't give me a fair shake. Discrimination feels like discrimination, even when it's for the best. My generation has been so socialized into our rights and so schooled away from discriminations of any kind, I didn't know how to be thankful. Thank you for stereotyping me. Thanks for excluding me from your violence, although I'm a relatively affluent tourist. Gratitude for being spared is something of a double bind. I wanted to lose. I wanted to lose like everybody else in order to keep that bit of dignity.

Somewhere there's a picture of my trip to New Orleans. Jane and I took a tour of the bayous on our last day. We'd heard about a guy named Sirus who operated a shrimp boat and ran a little tourist junket on the side. First he'd check his traps, then take you into the maze of ancient waterways where, at some point, he'd stop his big flat-bottomed boat and coax some alligators into the water. Marshmallows were his preferred bait. He also had a pet gator he brought with him on the trip. You could hold it.

I got on the boat and looked around for his pet but couldn't find its shape. That bothered me. A lot. The last thing I needed was to step on an alligator or to poke it with my cane. It was a big boat, though, with lots of benches, coils of rope stacked here and there, and all sorts of traps and equipment under tarps. The alligator could be anywhere.

Later, while the eight of us who'd paid for the trip ogled at the few alligators Sirus had coaxed from the banks, he walked behind the wheel of the boat, pulled away a blanket and picked up his five-foot long pet. I couldn't see what he carried, but I figured it out when the Texan woman next to me shrieked and launched into prayer. Apparently she hadn't read the whole brochure.

Sirus calmed her down and explained that the reptile was his pet. "Lady, she's a tame." He repeated, "Lady, she's a tame."

"But it looks so real!" the Texan exclaimed.

Pets are, for some, a set of unreal animals.

"She is real," Sirus said and tried to hand the gator to our praying Texan. She refused. Sirus turned to me. "How about you?" he asked. "You wanna hold her?"

Before I could answer, I had an alligator in my arms. The tail drooped down under its own weight. Sirus's pet felt like a bag of muscle. A very fine bag of muscle. It suffered the indignity of us all with an ancient patience I could only envy.

"Let me take a picture." Jane began to fumble with the camera.

I didn't want to betray how uncomfortable I felt, holding this thing, but the camera got it out of me. At home, Jane would describe the photo. She said that the alligator and I look like we're both smiling, but we aren't. We wanted to get our time together over with and do it before anybody got hurt.

So did Jane.

That Was There, This Is Here

People ask me what I hate most about blindness. A good answer would be blindness. I hate blindness most about blindness, but that's usually not what folks are after. Pick something, they say, something specific. Pushed to choose one big-time irritant, I'll go on the permanent record with public washrooms. They're a consistent disaster. On a good day, the public john for John Q. Public only proves, once and for all, hell is made of porcelain.

Let's say I've got a kindly waitress on my arm, one who's willing to make the long march with me. I know I should be relieved for the guiding hand, and I am, yet my gratitude is smothered by how excruciating it is, at the age of thirty-three, to have someone take me to the can. Maybe at seventy or eighty I could accept this as a fact of late life. We all hope the golden years will soften our pride, but I doubt it. Nonetheless, it's downright impossible to look and feel okay when, beyond the age of four, you must ask around for help with a potty trip.

But asking for help isn't what I worry about most these days. Getting through the door alone, that's the real pressure point.

The drama of approaching the men's room with a waitress on my arm is somewhat like a first date. At the door we're faced with the awkward problem of how to say goodbye, or whether we will. While I'm thanking her for the help, we'll both wonder if we'll shake hands and call it a night, no invitations inside this evening. Or, she will worry aloud, "Do you need me to follow you?" Or I will worry she's worried about this, and so on and so forth goes the neurotic ping-pong.

My anxiety is justified. I've learned there's no underestimating the verve with which some people will play Good Samaritan to the disabled. Even though I insist I don't need a hand beyond the door, sometimes this is mistaken for shyness or a silly desire not to be an imposition, particularly an imposition on a stranger who makes eight bucks an hour delivering burgers to tables, not blind men to urinals.

It's no problem, really, I assure her. Just point me in the right direction, I say, and send me in the room, white cane swinging. If nobody's in the men's room, I'll crash around and find the urinal myself. What I won't mention is that the only danger in going it alone is determining if I'm in front of a urinal or between two of them. I could feel for the layout with my cane, but a cane doesn't tell me if I'm connecting with the outside or inside edges. The best proof is in running a hand around whatever is in front of me. Just think about it.

I'm sorry to say, but that's where I draw the line. Admit it, you wouldn't run a hand around a urinal either. Standing in front of my best guess, I take my chances, and I'm sorry for the occasional misjudgment. You have to draw the line somewhere, preferably with a stick and not a finger.

Misjudgments remain a less humiliating prospect than the alternatives. Once a waiter dragged me by my arm through the door and into the washroom and swung me into an empty stall. "No need! No, there's no need," I pleaded, but he hauled me through the busy washroom with cheery assurances. I don't know what I did to deserve such kindness. It's hard to be snarky when someone is aiming for helpful. Yet, when he chirped, "Here you are. If you need anything else, I'll just be waiting right outside the door," who could possibly go?

When it comes to the men's room, I realize I'm doomed to a lifetime in the Freudian twilight zone of toilet training and independence. Most of the time, all I wanted was directions.

Once I asked for directions from a blurry red-headed waitress. She sidled up to my table's edge, surrounded by a perfumey fog. I began to fret. I was having a slow summer lunch at a Milestone's franchise in suburban Langley, my old hometown. More than usual I was hand-wringing about help to the men's room because, this being my hometown, I didn't know who might be watching or, worse, who my guiding waitress might be. What I did know was she wore a lot of the perfume aptly called Poison, and the scent gave me a double take.

Let me put an urban myth to rest. The myth of supersenses isn't true. When you're blind, your sense of smell does not, in my experience, rival Superman's. What happens is you make smell perform new, unconscious tasks, such as recognizing people. The brain may have previously given that function to sight, but new neural pathways grow between compensatory senses. In my daily comings and goings, a smell or a voice now evokes a friendly recognition for me as powerful as a distant profile or familiar face once did. Now that I'm blind, a smell can grab as it goes by, the way a glimpse could once snag my curiosity.

This waitress turned my head with the smell of Poison. Its sticky sweetness caught my attention like flypaper on my eyeball, tugging my nose towards her with recognition. The Poison told me I might be about to ask Heidi for washroom guidance.

Heidi was a legendary high school debutante who, back in grade eleven, only dated keggers, those jockish guys who loafed around basketball courts, drove convertible VW Cabriolets, and worked weekends singing fraternity versions of "Happy Birthday" at The Keg. Cosmic justice dictates that most should still be slinging lager there, but I'm sure most made out just fine in the dot-com boom. For some reason—a reason indigenous only to a John Hughes storyboard—Heidi took an interest in me for three weeks in grade eleven, much to every Polo-wearing boy's dismay, and much to my slack-jawed astonishment. Our match was, in high school paradigms, unnatural. Maybe her short-lived attraction to me was an impaired judgment caused by the chronic haze of Poison she wore. Who knows. Mine wasn't to question such a gift as her.

She dumped me after those blissful three weeks, and, what's worse, dumped me for a twenty-one-year-old security guard from Willowbrook Mall. He had an orange sports car and a moustache. I couldn't compete. Although Heidi and I were an unlawful match in the high school order, our breakup was highly orthodox. You are always dumped for someone you perceive to be your inferior. It allows you the cold comfort of calling rejection by its less painful name: injustice.

Now, here I was, years later, reawakened to my past humiliation, blind, and possibly about to ask Heidi for a tender hand to the commode.

"Would you like some more coffee?" asked the blur who might be her.

"I'd love some coffee, but I'd love to be in your washroom even more."

Yes, "creepy" is a good word for my attempt at a charming phrase.

"Uh, the men's room is just over that way," she said.

I stared vacantly ahead, and she, I imagine, continued to point wherever "that way" aimed. Then I heard the pleasant sound of coffee pouring.

"I'm sorry," I interrupted. "I don't know what that means. I don't know what that way means." I plucked my white cane from the bag beside me. "See?" I showed her. "I guess it wasn't obvious, and I forgot to mention—"

"Oh my god! I'm so sorry, I didn't know you were blind! You didn't look—You don't look. . . . Not at all, really."

I smiled with that warm feeling you get when you're sixteen and someone says you look like you're in your twenties. Maybe it wouldn't be so awful to run into Heidi after all.

"Thanks, that's very kind. Where'd you say that washroom is?"

"Oh, right. The men's room is at the back."

"Where's the back?"

"Over there," she said, and walked away.

All I wanted were directions, but, instead, my waitress had pointed to the blind spots in language. They'd eroded at some point along with my eyesight. In the nature of blind spots, I hadn't noticed this new one, until she pointed to it.

You could say my waitress diagnosed a condition in language parallel to the one my doctor had found in my retinas. My peripheral vision was almost gone, and language's ability to point and refer had narrowed, too. Those bits of language are over there, that way. Some are right here, in front of you. Here. No, here. Right there, in the way we speak.

What's odd, though, is they are not the elements of language most blind people prickle about. Usually blind militants tub-thump about the sight-centred features of English idiom. Look at you! What a sight you are! A real looker. And you're a vision. Beauty is in the eye of the beholder. So nice to see you! Things looking up? I've had my eye on you, so I looked into it, kept my eyes peeled, and here you are, a sight for sore eyes, but no eyesore. Out of sight! What have you got your sights on these days? Look out! Watch it! Be on the lookout, keep your eye on the ball. I'll see to it. See you later? See you around. See?

On the flip side, English encourages the use of derogative blindness metaphors to mean things other than "without sight." Some of these connotations include ignorant, limited, deranged, deceived, terminal, stupid, false, naïve, and, of course, confused.

But visual and blind metaphors have never bothered me. You won't hear my fist slamming a podium about my victimization at the hands of metaphors or our tendency to assume sightedness. I once bought some cologne at a department store. As I caned by, the man at the counter stopped me to give his sales pitch.

"The fabulous feature of this elegant cologne is that you can keep it in the freezer and refresh yourself on a hot summer day with a stimulating, cool blast of aromatic body spray."

Kinky, I thought. I'll take it. He asked if I'd like to look at the swishy design of the bottle, then held it up for me to inspect.

"See the lovely edging?" he asked.

I couldn't tell where the bottle went, so I stood there, waving my hand around trying to find where he'd hoisted the glassy smear. Realizing his mistake, the salesman smacked himself repeatedly on the forehead with his palm, muttering "stupid, stupid, stupid." That was unnecessary, and perhaps as embarrassing for me as it was for him.

These features of the language truly don't bother me because they are metaphors and I understand them that way. They still mean something to me, too, probably because I saw once. But I don't see any need to make a big fuss about them now. Next thing you know, we'll demand the sound "eye" be removed from "blind." From that we'll achieve the significant political success of becoming blond as a bat or blended by the light. Or maybe just bland.

My waitress's words of guidance are the true linguistic peculiarity, one worth paying attention to. This, that, there, here, and so on, the indexicals that are used to point—

literally—beyond the page or the speaker's finger, have lost their meaning for me, the hands of the words chopped off by my narrowing field of vision.

I'm surprised that blindness can alter language and permanently disable parts of speech. My words, it would appear, are part of my body, and can suffer the pathology of its diseases as well.

"Excuse me."

My waitress was back, and not a second too late to take another crack at directions.

"I don't mean to intrude," she said, "but didn't you go to Langley Secondary School?"

The future flashed. Jeering keggers point and snicker as Heidi tows me off to the washroom. A security guard with a big-ass moustache waits for us at the men's room and says, "I'll take him from here, honey."

"Yes, yes, I did go to Langley Secondary."

"I thought so! It's Ryan, right? I'm Danielle! We were in drama class together. God, I didn't recognize you at all."

The fists I've balled in my lap relax. I can feel the natural slouch of my spine returning. The Poison takes on a slightly different sweetness.

"You look so different now," she said.

Blindness can have that effect, I thought, and braced myself.

"You too," I replied, then realized how utterly confusing that must be.

"I'm not sure what it is. Maybe it's because—"

The blank stare? The fierce squint? The face of disorientation?

"It's—well . . ." She placed her hand on my head with daring compassion. "I know! You shaved your head. When did you do that?"

I burned with a new embarrassment at my narcissism. Just because it's a sighted world, blindness doesn't have to be the first thing people see.

"I remember back in high school, your hair used to be really long, at least down to here."

"Yes," I smiled, "to here."

I'll Be Waiting

These two drunks are having an argument outside a bar.
They were arguing as to whether that object up in the sky
was the sun or the moon. A third drunk stumbles out of the
bar, and one of them walks up to him and says, "Buddy,
will you help us out? We're in an argument, and we can't
decide who's right." The third drunk asks, "What's the
argument?" "We want to know, 'Is that the sun or the moon
up there?'" The third drunk says, "Aw, I dunno, man.
I ain't from this neighbourhood."

—as told by Townes Van Zandt

In the autumn of 1995, a few months after Jane and I parted
ways, I enrolled as a graduate student in the English
Department at Simon Fraser University. I could still read, but
barely. At most I could see three letters of a word at once. For
my course of study, my eyes gravitated me towards poetry. The
briefer, the better. I also took courses in children's literature,
appreciating the really, really short words. Because of the extra
time reading demanded and because of the split with Jane, I
decided I would focus all my energy on my studies. Not two
days into the semester, I met a woman named Tracy.

She had moved to Vancouver from the prairies. Tall and fair, with dark brown hair and a pixie-like face, she turned our heads. The newbie graduate boys followed her around campus, all of us cloying for attention. She suffered our charms with a wry grin on her face and sometimes egged us on. Maybe she looked over her shoulder as she walked away from us or touched our arms as she passed. Whatever Tracy did, it made us crazy.

My office was across the hall from hers. Luckily for me, we both smoked. Her office had a balcony, but mine didn't. I knocked on her door one afternoon and asked if I could borrow her ledge. To smoke, I assured her. She joined me outside. Soon I stopped by often, and soon I inhaled about twice as many cigarettes as normal.

"I was thinking," I said one day, "maybe you and I should do something sometime. It's my birthday next weekend. I thought maybe—"

"I can't," she said flatly.

"Alrighty then. That's okay, I understand."

"Because it's my birthday, too," she finished.

We'd been born twelve hours apart. Having discovered that, we hung around together the rest of the day until, finally, she insisted that she had some work to finish. A pile of notes needed keyboarding, and the computer workroom would be too busy soon.

"Are you fast at typing?" I asked.

"I'm okay."

"Because I can type, like, fifty words a minute. I mean, I'd be happy to burn through your stuff, and then, I dunno,

107

maybe we could go eat or something." I was already an hour late for a seminar about a book I hadn't read.

"You don't have to do that," she said. "I'll get it done at my own pace."

"But I'm really fast. Greased lightning. It would save you a lot of time, and then we could go do something."

"Really, you don't have to do that for me."

"But I insist."

Tracy let me type while she reclined in a chair and dictated her notes. I explained that keyboarding was the best thing I'd learned in high school. I didn't need to look. I could feel what I was doing. The difference saved me a lot of grief. I encouraged her to learn the skill, too, if she had time. She listened and agreed and, all the while, knew she could type faster than two of me.

Not long before, Tracy had separated from her boyfriend of many years. Our shared recognition—an immediate and unspoken one—that we could fall hard and long for each other was a bit too much so soon. Both of us still wanted a few lost weekends and compensatory trysts. We dated but agreed to leave the playing field open, neither of us ready for a serious thing.

I had only one difficulty with our arrangement. Tracy casually dated a few guys, while I wooed, well, her. It wasn't for lack of trying, either, especially after one of her new beaus, a long-haired, revolutionary wannabe, tried to convince Tracy to give me the shrug-off. According to her macho cupcake, I was all brains, no physicality. For a degenerating blind guy, it was a bitter shot of neurotic juice. He thrust me into competition. I found myself running in the alpha Olympics of male sexuality, without prowess or dignity. I intended to make Tracy as jealous as I was, if not more.

Desire. The word itself originates from Sirius, the guiding star, a fixed and heavenly point of light. We navigate the world by it, and in relationship to that star, we know our place. This image, the source of the word's meaning, is true to my experience. The feeling of desire not only directs us but compels us forward. We are, as they say, moved by desire.

Also implied is that desire remains a point of no arrival, a permanently remote idea we follow, and follow some more. As one might imagine, blindness doesn't cooperate well with guidance from stars, suns, moons, or light bulbs. Anything light-oriented, really. At the time, I could still glimpse the tiniest bit of what I desired, but that didn't guarantee I knew where the hell I was going.

During my university years, I had a favourite watering hole. The pub was called the Rose and Thorn but was known to its regulars more evocatively by its acronym, the Rat. When I was an undergraduate student, I often hung out there and read novels, even sketched outlines for papers on my napkin, or made notes on my expired bus transfers. The rest of the time, I tried to look artsy. For me, the Rat was an oddly productive joint. Once, before heading off to fall down in nightclubs, I spent a beery evening there with *The Sun Also Rises*. More than the book, I remember my accompanying fixation. I wanted to finish my first Hemingway novel with a pickled egg and an existential crisis on a mechanical bull. Neither was an option at the Rat, although it seemed like the kind of place you'd find personal growth through a mechanical bull or competitive patron tossing. I settled for a pack of Doritos and change for the bus to my next stop. Modern literature is always better with accessories, if you can find them.

Tonight Tracy was out on the town with one of her courting beaus. I figured if I was going to spend some quality time with my thoughts, why not take them out to the Rat. At least in a pub, the public had some chance of finding me. If I couldn't read a novel there anymore, not under the poor lighting, at least I might find myself in a story. That was my thinking, if you could call it that.

One of the many things blindness makes me forget is that I still have to put my eyes somewhere. Daydreaming or listening to the music or conversations around me, I don't lend enough attention to where I may have placed my gaze for the past five or ten minutes. When in public, I would be wise to screw my eyes to the table or floor, but I forget they're casting about, saying things like, "Hello there," or, "Hey, don't I know you?" Or any number of accidental messages. Because I may not recognize what's across the room, wherever I've locked my cattle stare, sometimes I inadvertently enter a staring contest with strangers who, unaware of my blindness, peg me for either an apprenticing hypnotist, a vacant psychopath, or, worse, a poorly socialized lech.

I knew I'd goofed up when I heard footsteps march towards me, high-heeled steps clicking louder and louder as they approached. The confident stride didn't alarm me so much as the halting sound, a brief, accusatory silence that parked beside my table. The shadowy blur of a woman wanted to know what I thought I was staring at. So did I. It took me a few beats to manage a guess.

"Uh, nothing? I was just looking at, well, no, nothing, really."

"Well, I don't know what's fascinating you so much," she said, "but, if you don't mind, my friend and I over there would appreciate it if you'd stop staring at us and our, uh, nothing. Frankly, it's fucking creepy."

Saying that I saw "nothing" was untrue. I could have sworn, from across the room, that the profile of her head had been a poster. A poster of a beer mug. I didn't think that would please her, so I kept it to myself.

I confabulate images all the time. They can get me into trouble, too. Unoccupied or restless, my eyes make up things to see, things constructed from what little information they still receive. Sometimes the blind claim to see bits of the immediate world, perhaps a person they are talking to, with extraordinary detail and complexity. It isn't a memory of an image but a fresh and animated vision that feels, as only sight can, that it is real, not emerging from your mind and its still-active eye. It is phantom sight. And then it is gone, as fast as it came. Sometimes the image morphs into another vivid con-fabulation. A black garbage bag on the floor becomes a slick puddle of oil. Then, when I touch it, I feel the bundled black leather coat I'm looking for. Likelihood plays a role. I don't mistake mailboxes for jigging leprechauns, but sometimes I can mistake, say, a woman sitting against a wall for a poster of a beer mug. I thought her blond hair was foam.

Under the table, my white cane remained on the floor, out

of sight. My accuser hadn't detected my blindness. I was passing for sighted, so although she was pissed, I was mildly pleased. In this circumstance arises a difficult choice. I have to decide whether I'm going to let my condition hang out, which can embarrass that person and cause them to retreat, or whether I'm going to continue to pass for sighted, which is sometimes an easier option for us both.

A moment like that one has a writerly craft. That is, I have to guess at the possible scope of my story with someone, and quickly. If I don't think we'll become bosom buddies, if I don't think I'll ever meet this person again, I'll often try to pass for sighted. I do that because I don't want to field their discomfort and because I'd prefer not to give my spiel about what I can and can't see, what caused it, and so on. Meanwhile, the person lets their embarrassment deflate. If I say I'm blind, though, in my mind I've made a gesture of desire, even a small one, to keep alive the possibility for some sustained relationship, risking their embarrassment as a cost.

It's a conundrum every time. If I'm honest, people often hightail it, but if I lie, they're more likely to hang around and discover the lie.

"I'm sorry," I decided to say, "I was just kind of daydreaming, and these are my old glasses, so I guess I didn't notice I was staring at you. Sorry about that. I didn't mean to creep anybody out. Not that I know of."

She laughed, albeit slightly. I moved my foot under the table to check my cane. Everything from tip to handle was sufficiently out of sight, or so I thought. As apology for the creep factor, I asked if my accuser and her friend would join me for a drink, which she accepted, with some reluctance. When she went to fetch her friend, I snatched my cane from under the table, collapsed it to its bundle of segments and stuffed the works into my satchel. So much anxiety over so little, I know, but there it was, my blindness packed away like the tidy stack of dynamite it is. If I was going to pass for sighted, at least for a while, I didn't want either of them to feel my cane under their feet and have to deal with, hey, how did that white cane get there? I wonder where the poor blind person is who left that behind?

It happens, too. I've left my cane all over the city, prompting hundreds of speculations about my own whereabouts and survival. It's easy to lose a cane. It's as easy as losing a pair of glasses or looking through the glasses on your nose and wondering where you could have left them this time. Pick up two grocery bags, one in each hand, and, voila, you forget your cane on the bus bench. Believe it or not, the principal cause is routine. I forget I'm blind all the time, even when I'm bumping around with extra difficulty. The cane, like blindness or even my gaze, becomes such a habitual part of life's rhythm that each is easily disregarded. Losing a cane can even happen despite a person's best efforts.

The most stylish case I know of happened to my only blind friend, Willy. Once he tried to get on the Skytrain, Vancouver's gaudy monorail, when the doors closed as he was about to board. The two doors snapped shut, stranding Willy on the platform. His white cane remained partially on board, clenched between the doors like a toothpick between teeth. Willy yanked and yanked, but the doors were too tight.

Within seconds the train departed and dragged Willy's aid along with it, the cane narrowly missing passengers waiting on the platform as it swept by like a scythe. That must have looked neat. I've often wondered what people at the next station thought when the doors opened and an ownerless white cane dropped at their feet.

If I couldn't control my blindness, at least I could control its introduction. If anything, I figured I would reveal my condition to my new acquaintances later, if the circumstance demanded it. I had to hope I wouldn't need the washroom anytime soon. If we got along and we were all comfortable and affable with one another, my blindness would be a surprise, maybe even a mysterious facet of character. A man can daydream. I might stand up to pay the bill, retrieve my cane, and snap it open with veteran grace, only to astonish the table with my casual delivery. My god, they would gasp. We had no idea you were . . . you are. . . . To that I would feign an endearing humbleness. Oh, you mean this, this cane? It's nothing, really. Oh my, how I always forget about my blindness. I guess it's just one of those things. A mysterious facet of character, perhaps.

That would be nice. More likely, though, I would get up to pay the bill, open my stick, and poke one of my new acquaintances in the forehead. She would be surprised and bleeding, but more surprised at the coldness of the beers I'd then knock over as I turned to apologize. Then I'd elbow somebody in the face, or everybody. Noses would break as I bulled my way out of the booth. That would be more my style. After paying the bill, I would also return to the wrong table, seduce the empty chairs, and my two victims would take that opportunity to make for the nearest exit. Not that I want to elicit pity. Blindness, no matter how traumatizing, is a constant state of slapstick. Sometimes the innocent have to go down with me.

By this time in my pathology, I'd passed for sighted on many occasions, even daily, but in short intervals involving little movement. Sitting in a booth and chit-chatting is close to still life. I reasoned passing shouldn't be too hard. No forklifts, no Louisiana muggers, and no complicated zippers were here to contend with. All would be fine. I simply had to work at general eye contact and keep my hand on my beer at all times. Let go of that, and I'd grope around the table, pinching the air like a dumb crab. The trick is to focus people on what I'm saying, not what I'm doing. And keep all movements to a minimum, no matter what.

The conversation did play out well, after all, and I never did reveal my blindness. Nobody seemed the wiser. Passing for sighted can be fun when it works, although not entirely relaxing. It's a kind of holiday, though, hanging out with normalcy. I groused about skiing accidents, road trips, and other visual experiences I either updated from my sighted days or stole from my sighted friends. Most of the time, the art of passing depends on an intimacy with my own nostalgia. Otherwise it requires access to bullshit drowned in persuasive detail.

"Yeah, I've seen my share of crappy jobs, too," I recalled at one point. "I had a job a few summers ago at, um, what's it called? The wheat, the wheat something. The wheat? Shit, it's gone."

"Was it a bakery?" asked the woman who'd accused me of staring.

"No. Where all the wheat is transferred, down by the waterfront."

"The Wheat Transfer?" asked her friend.

"No. It's like—"

"The Wheat Dock?"

"No, no, it's like collection, like wheat hoarding or something. I can't—"

My accuser enjoyed that. "The Wheat Collection Agency?" she said. "Did you rough people up for their bad wheat debts or something? Were you, like, a repo-man for wheat farmers?" She laughed, and I liked the sound of it.

"Yes, I had a gun, and I took back borrowed wheat—at the Wheat Pool! That's what it's called. The Wheat Pool. Anyways, seriously, I was actually a bin picker there."

"What's a bin picker?" my accuser asked.

A bin picker was the most interesting job I knew, and one I'd never worked. My friend Wayde had been hired to it the summer after high school. It had always struck me as the strangest job, and I thought it made a good story. For five years I'd been a student. Not much hilarity or anecdotal thrill comes of nights with a broken spell-check.

"A bin picker is a person who hangs in empty grain silos. I wore, like, a nylon harness and they strung me from a winch. We wore goggles and air masks because it was so dirty. Our job was to chip the silo walls clean with a pickaxe. Or a hoe. Something like that. Anyways, I whacked all the grain off, whatever stuff stuck to the insides, just hanging in the air like

that for hours. Really suffocating stuff. Crummy work.
Maybe as lousy as the summer I drove a forklift. God, I hate
forklifts."

By the end of the night, my accuser had softened up to me.
We seemed more than happy with each other's company.
Neither of us wanted to call it quits at closing time, so when
her friend was off buying a bag of chips, my accuser asked me
if I wanted to meet back at her place later. The pub had
worked, for once. I had been found by the public. My story,
and storytelling, were going places I hadn't planned. Such is
desire's guidance, sometimes.

"Just give me a half an hour to drop my friend off," she
said, putting her jacket on. She wrote an address on a coaster
and slid it into my shirt pocket.

"I'll see you there," I said.

"I'll be waiting."

Finding her apartment wasn't a problem. I gave the coaster
to my cab driver and let him do the reading and the navigating. I knew I was in a bit of an awkward position, though,
having withheld the whole blindness thing far too long. After
all the stories I'd pinched from my friends' lives, too, it would
be extra hard now to comfortably retrofit my life as anything
other than theatre. I reasoned, with a boozy, horny compul-
sion, I'd best just keep up the sighted routine indefinitely.
Why ruin a perfectly good night? When I reached her apartment building, I imagined I would be able to cane my way to
the door without her spotting me. I hoped. Once inside, I'd
find her apartment in the lit hallways, fold my cane back into
my satchel, knock on the door, and wing it from there.

Couches are easy to find in apartments. If I'd entered and she'd asked me to find the TV remote, that would be game over.

What can I say in my defence? Nothing. How can I explain all this duplicity? Desperation might be a start, and basic reptilian instinct, I guess, anything to earn the desire of another. If I dig a bit deeper, though, the more interesting answer is that I would, at that time, have done anything not to appear blind. Sacrificing self-respect was a minor casualty. I couldn't cure blindness in myself, so I was doing my best to make a man and a life that excluded it as long as possible. It was a form of self-medication. Lies masked and deferred my symptoms. Sometimes.

When the cabbie pulled up to the building, I asked what number I was looking for. He said 107, and handed me back my golden coaster. I got out of the cab, under a bright streetlight, and looked around, unable to make out the blocky features I attribute to an apartment building. No grids of light hung in the sky to suggest apartments, not even one with an I'll-be-waiting light in the window.

Before I shut the car door, I asked, "Where's the entrance?"

"Which one?" the driver said.

"What do you mean? To the building."

"To 107? Man, I don't know. The path here is sort of an entrance. Follow the sidewalk to your left, and your address is somewhere in there."

"Okay. Thanks."

"Do you want me to guide you?"

"No," I lied for the last time. "I'm fine."

I shut the door, turned, then walked directly into a large bush. The cabbie rolled his window down and coached me further to the left. I felt a sidewalk under my cane. The concrete lead away from the street, but to what, I couldn't tell.

"The townhouses are just down there," he said, and drove away.

The evening air felt cool on my face and refreshed my senses after the smoky bar and musty cab. All was silence except for the buzz of streetlights. The sound diminished behind me as I walked into what I now assumed was a townhouse complex. I caned my way along the main concrete footpath, tapping the edges to know my position and tapping the middle to ensure a clear way. I tried to create as little noise as possible, but it was hard to muffle each strike. Soon, when I did tap, I could hear the sound change, echoing off what were buildings, townhouses, on either side. In the new tone I could hear the deepening enclosure around me. At the end of each house's walkway was a small, decorative lantern, each of them dimly lit. The pattern suggested a horseshoe of houses, none of them illuminated, none of them enumerated in any way I could see.

Quietly I made my way to one of the darkened doors and felt for information. A mail slot and peephole, a little arched window, I recognized those, but no numbers. Back to the main walkway I retreated and approached the next house, again palming about in hopes of a raised number. Most people in the complex, I could only assume, didn't want to be found. Could be a witness protection housing project. Maybe the next door would be numbered.

When my fingertips felt the wood of the third door, a dog exploded into voice on the other side. I thought I could taste adrenaline. Mass market production kicked in, heavy distribution, too. Then my body shifted from startled to fully alarmed when the animal threw its weight, repeatedly, at the hinged bit of wood between us. The dog had its own desires, and my flesh was on its wish list. A man's voice bellowed from inside.

"Otto!! Otto, no! Ott-o, shut up or you're glue!"

On my next try, I picked a darkened door that just happened to sport a set of raised numbers nailed above the peephole. 1-0-3, I felt, so I counted four decorative lanterns down the walkway, and approached 107 at last. Again I palmed the door and the surrounding wall. No number confirmed the address. Fuck it, I thought, how could this be anything but 107? 103 plus 4 is 107. The math doesn't lie.

Unless they're duplexes. I did the new math. Being about three o'clock in the morning, and several pints past reasonable, it took me a minute to come up with number 111 as the other possible address I was about to wake. I debated what to do next. More hand-to-door number research didn't appeal. Instead, I tried my last covert option. The door handle. It turned.

Caution and propriety are resources of character I do call upon. Not often enough, maybe. For a few moments I puzzled at the handle, wondering if it was meant for me or if it was the most unfortunate temptation I would know in my short life. And where would that life go from here? Prison on breaking and entering charges? Would a judge buy my plea of poor math and dying retinas? Or maybe I was about to enter a house of vigilante justice, its owners educated by the old copies of *Guns & Ammo* stacked on the coffee table. Then I heard my intended's phrase in my ear again. "I'll be waiting," she said. Could this open door be what she meant? Was it some sort of friendly, trusting gesture or, better, some sort of playful kink? Was she really waiting, I mean, really waiting, somewhere in the house, for me to breeze in and assume some sort of role play? I was born in Langley. I don't know these things.

I opened the door a crack and poked my head inside. "Hello?"

Nobody answered. I tried again, a little louder. Nobody answered.

My cue to go home couldn't be more plain. This was either the wrong house, or my new acquaintance had passed out as a lady-in-waiting. Either way, nothing good would come of this. Meanwhile, I'd already stepped inside to nose around.

At first I wasn't sure what to do with the door. When one breaks into a house, should one leave the door open for a quick getaway, or should one close it for a modicum of privacy? I left it open. When I was caught, it would support my claim I was just leaving.

My impulse was to flick a light on, so I wiped the walls with my hands, like Marcel Marceau in search of a switch. As I felt about, I discovered a little side table tucked near the door, up against the wall. I pawed the surface for a lamp, unable to find one. A short stack of mail revealed itself to my hand, three envelopes with plastic windows. I snatched the lot and left, shutting the door behind me. Now I could add theft to my growing list of charges, which probably wouldn't do anything to bolster my prison rep. And what a rep it would be.

"Whatcha in for?" my new cellmate would ask. In his hand would be a toothbrush, the one he was sharpening against our cell wall.

"Theft," I'd say, puffing with pride.

For a moment my new cellmate, Critter or Elmo or The Crank, or whatever his name is, he would stop production on his new shank and turn to inspect me, the new fish.

"Oh yeah? Whadja get?"

I'd say, "Two to five on a bum beef," and hope to sound schooled in the lingo of the clink.

"What the fuck's a bum beef? I meant whadja get, whadja steal, fish."

"Fish? No, can't say I got a fish," I'd admit, "although I did catch a trout once. I didn't have a licence, either."

"No, no!" he'd bellow, as if commanding his old dog, Otto. "You, you're a fish, that's what a fish is, a new guy. Get it?" Each of his phrases would finish with a little jab of the tooth-brush in my direction. "Whadja really get, fish?"

"Do you mean what did I steal?"

"Okay, whadja steal?"

"A phone bill."

"A phone bill?"

"Yeah. Oh, and a chance to win millions, but I never got a chance to open it."

With my incriminating evidence in hand, I retreated to the street and its buzzing lights. There I held up the mail and tried to read the addresses in the little windows. The streetlight, no better than the lamps in the ambient Rat, was either too dim, or it glanced off the plastic and obliterated anything legible. Back to the unknown townhouse I caned my way.

As I walked, I gave myself a stern talking to. Slide the envelopes back through the slot and call it a night. Get out while you can, I advised. I agreed with myself. I returned the mail through the mail slot and, ready to go home, stood up straight, opened the door, and walked inside for another look around.

If a cause for my situation could be anything other than desire, I'd blame my night on grain silos. Getting lost inside a townhouse was poetic punishment for my own deceptions. I was wandering in the dark, bumping into somebody's TV, then their couch, and then some thing sharp and rigid on the floor I couldn't identify. In effect, I was a man aimlessly picking at the edges of a ridiculous, empty deception. One with a staircase, I discovered.

As I felt my way back to the door, ready to go home, I happened upon a bottom step which, I assumed, led up to the bedrooms.

Up the stairs I crept, slowly, painfully, one creaking step at a time. I came to the landing. The landing was good. And on the seventh day, when I reached the top step, I rested. I listened. Not a sound, which could be the sound of somebody waiting, the right somebody, I hoped. The air smelled of hotdogs. I took a step into the hallway. Down I planted my boot on something soft. A doll wailed under my foot.

Without thinking, I grabbed the toy and stuffed it into my satchel. That seemed the most expedient way to suffocate it, but my bag wasn't enough. Down the stairs I ran, then bolted out the front door, with doll-child crying.

The ride was over, I'd been nicely tossed, and I'd had enough. I resolved to go home, if I could find it. Under no circumstance was I going back inside to replace the doll. I removed it from my satchel and left it on the doormat.

Who knows if I was in the right house that night. My lady in waiting hadn't mentioned a child or a kid brother or sister, but then again I hadn't mentioned a few details of my own. On the coaster she'd given me was an address but no phone number. In the sober light of morning, I felt no temptation to navigate my way back. Instead, I phoned Tracy. She was home and hoping I would call. We talked for hours over breakfast, as if in the same kitchen. It was one of many dates to come.

I like to imagine a family getting up that morning, and one of them opening the front door to fetch the newspaper. Next to it is the doll, asleep on the front steps, like a drunk who didn't make it all the way home. Nobody can figure it out. Perhaps little Cathy left her Wailing Hazel on the porch yesterday. Or maybe Cathy's dad, Critter, dropped it while unloading the family monster truck. Or maybe the doll is given the mystery it deserves, like some ownerless white cane left at the station.

The Pusan Roach

"Batman?" I asked. "Is Batman here?"

Children darted back and forth across my tunnel vision. Again I hailed Batman, louder this time, with a little more authority in my tone.

"Everybody stop, please, please stop. I'm looking for Batman."

It occurred to me that I might never utter this phrase again, not without straps and a gurney holding me down.

It was my first day teaching in South Korea. Among other things, I could hear lips sputtering like the engines of cars and planes, a soundtrack for the ongoing chases around the room. Only a couple of kids sat around a large, yellow table and quietly disappeared into their stashes of paper and pens. So far, roll call involved nobody but me.

As a boy flew by, I caught his elbow. Maybe I was in the wrong room. Taped to the door, an illustration of a piece of fruit identified each class. In my eyes, though, an apple could be a strawberry. The globby smear looked red, but that's about it. I couldn't even be certain of the colour.

"Is this Apple Class?" I asked and pointed to the drawing.

"Apple teach-ah! You Apple teach-ah!" he agreed.

"Yes, good. Do you know who Batman is?"

"Batman!" he agreed, and performed some superhero gestures. That's what I thought I saw. Maybe he suffered a violent tic. I couldn't tell.

"Okay, Batman, I'm Ryan."

"Lion?" He was ecstatic. "Lion teach-ah! Lion King!" He growled, roared, then swiped my thigh with an imaginary paw.

Because teaching English was my new job in Pusan, I made my first attempt to concern myself with Batman's pronunciation, confident, however, that I really couldn't care less.

"No, not Lion. R-r-ryan. R-r-ryan. See? Now you try."

As he ran away, he belted out my name.

"R-r-r-r-l-lion King teach-ah Lion the King his teach!"

Both Tracy and I had arrived in Pusan late the previous night. At 7:30 the next morning, I took charge of my first students, gobsmacked and clueless what to do. Had I the resources, Apple Class would be bobbing for Ritalin after roll call. No such luck. I didn't know any educational games, either. A few promising titles came to mind. "Which Plant Am I?" suited my pace, or, better, we could play "Sleep Clinic."

Schooling a kid named Batman was a surprise, and it wasn't. I say I taught English in South Korea, but that's too noble a job description. Really I made American cultural products and franchise crud more accessible. It didn't take long to figure out. Waiting on my desk, next to the class list, was a textbook. The first chapter focused on a movie called *Dinosaur Park*. It wasn't an ad, of course, no, but a helpful narrative about, what else, verbs. Giant lizards, both extinct and resurrected, need a constant supply of past tense. Add the Lion King and Batman to that English class. Somebody's native culture was losing to the usual superpowers, kaplowy and hakuna matata.

Of the little Korea Tracy and I had encountered so far, much declared the firm economic presence of the west. Everything was familiar but new, mistranslated, and garbled, as if we'd moved overseas to live in a nifty satire of America. As we drove from the airport, Tracy saw restaurants with English names in neon, everything from Bone to Poem to Smog. I, for one, loved to grog at Smog. Forgotten Hollywood personalities crowded billboards with their big white teeth. According to Tracy, Meg Ryan seemed especially popular. Meg's face adorned the city enough that we had to wonder if she'd led a coup.

Postered about the streets were ads for bands, too. Tracy rattled off some names as we drove by. I'd forgotten most of the groups long ago, along with any desire to wear sweatbands or cock-rock iron-on shirts. Kam-sa-ham-ni-da, South Korea! We are the Scorpions, and we rocked you like a hurricane! Maybe they taught English on the side. Everybody relied on the industry enough.

Then came the images of some older, other Korea, the one being edged out. Tracy described the scenes to me. She saw squat neighbourhood temples between international banks, sidewalk noodle and soju tents in front of Subway, and, between megamalls, the slender alleyway entrances to original public markets, their fresh fish and eel aquariums stacked like retainer walls against brightly painted chain stores.

All this in one night's drive from the airport. Arriving at our new home, a sign and a fence warned about the undetonated landmines in the neighbouring hillside.

This isn't to say Pusan lacked its own modernity. Taking in the neighbourhood on our first morning, Tracy and I passed groups of high school students who sported pink, furry, over-sized gloves, purses, puffy jackets, and aviator helmets. The candy-floss look belonged to a new Korean tweeny band called H.O.T., or High-Five of Teenagers. Dig it. A spiffy style, some would say, although far more suitable to snowy northern British Columbia than a country with punitive humidity. Still, the puffy gloves were handy. My older students begged to shammy the chalkboard with them, or, if need be, with their jackets and purses and hats, everybody rubbing their wardrobes against the day's English.

Even the soundscape gave new meaning. My first morning began with a garbage truck bleating opera through a scratchy megaphone. Tracy and I lived in a renovated office several floors above the school. From our bedroom window, she watched our neighbours scramble roadside with their trash and receive a fresh roll of toilet paper in return.

Overseas, in all these extremes of the familiar and the new, I would test my relationship to blindness and Tracy. Here I would become a caricature of myself by exhausting the limits of my sight and my denial. My brother, Mykol, had foreshadowed the problem well. As a going-away present, he made me a card. Cartooned on the front was a bald, spectacled, and gangly Ryan, pigeon-toed and squinty. On the chalkboard behind me, my name appeared as only I write it. All four letters were different sizes, scattered, and at different heights on the board. That's what happens when you see as little as I did then. Batman and I had something in common already. We were both imported cartoons, and, most worrisome, I too had a secret identity. For the next six months, I would pretend I could see.

Now that I'd found Batman, I returned to the roll call. My micro-island of good sight dropped down a line and revealed the next name two letters at a time. Another Batman. I checked the next name, and the next, and counted four more to go. The roll call wasn't alphabetical. Below the Batmans bulged a pile of five Arnolds. A dull ache began behind my eyes from reading. Adding to it was the noise, the firefly movements of children, the jet lag, and the immediacy of my situation. How would I manage all of this with such dismal eyesight? What was I thinking when I signed on for manic seven year olds? I honestly hadn't considered my body among theirs, not until reality flew around the room making car and airplane noises.

I called the next Batman, but nobody answered. Because pleading didn't work, I trawled the room with my arms open like a fishnet. Finally, with all twenty kids corralled around the yellow table, we got down to who was who, and who I would be.

Ours was a specialty private institution called a *hagwan*. Extra school, you might say. We taught English, math, and arts, employing local teachers, except Tracy and me, the expats. Our two positions were most of the branding and marketing, a couple of western white faces smiling on the school's brochure. Such faces suggested we don't just teach English here, we teach real English, the kind that passes through glossy North American lips. The kind of lips Meg Ryan uses. Upon enrollment, everybody adopted his or her favourite English name. Fantasy Island never offered so much.

Along with the Batmans and Arnolds, all of whom were reborn as Batman or Arnold One through Five, I taught bouquets of Lilies, Daisies, and Roses. I taught gangs of video game characters, a few hopeful Meg Ryans, an equal number of Michael Jacksons, and even a couple of Kevins, as in Costner. Those kids had sat through the Robin Hood flick a few too many times. When I called their names, each said, "Here, teach-ah!" then perforated me with imaginary arrows.

Between the two Kevins on my Apple Class list, I found what I thought was a lost third.

"Cabin?" I called.

"Here, teach-ah!" he replied, then stood up on his chair and shot me.

"Thank you."

I checked the list again. The previous teacher had spelled the name just the way I'd said it.

"Do you mean you want the name Kevin, Cabin?"

I said each name slowly and exaggerated the difference. I still didn't care one way or the other, but since I didn't know what else to do with my class, Cabin's name seemed a good enough pastime as any.

"No," he said. "Cabin."

"Cabin Costner?"

"Yes, teach-ah."

"You mean Kevin, Cabin."

"No, teach-ah, Cabin, Ca-bin."

His impatience was noted. Before I took another arrow, I asked a girl next to me for help. "May I use your pen and paper?"

She grinned fiercely, as if her pigtails pulled the smile out of her face. I slid her materials my way, sketched a log cabin, then held it up for everyone to see.

"A cabin," I explained, then wrote the word under the picture. "This is a cabin." I added the name Kevin and held it up again, trying to enunciate the difference. "Cabin, Kevin, Cabin, Kevin. See? Cabin, you mean Kevin, right?"

Nobody made a sound.

I wondered if maybe my cabin didn't look like one at all. I could only make out bits of it myself. Maybe it looked like lumber or wieners in a package, if Pusan grocers sold wieners in a package. I didn't know. Or maybe it looked like a tidy pile of shit. Cabin finally ventured a different guess.

"Teach-ah is, um," he pointed to the drawing, "Lion teach-ah's house?"

My good eye, the one that still had tunnel vision, surveyed the table. Slowly I cobbled together twenty blank and puzzled stares.

In that moment, a new pedagogy, my pedagogy as an ambassador for the English language, was born. I decided, for better or for worse, as long as I taught in South Korea, I would go along with anything my kids fancied.

I say I taught English in South Korea, but from that moment on it was my English, not the Queen's and not

Disney's. Scrabble quickly became the standard teaching tool and laboratory for my technique. A typical class would soon unfold something like this.

"Teach-ah," Meg Ryan Two might ask. "What is—?" She'd point to the Scrabble board at the word she'd made but couldn't pronounce.

Let's say the letters K, P, I and Q were strategically placed with the Q on a double-letter score. First I would scan the board for whatever Meg had pointed at, and feign deep thought while my good eye searched. Once I found the word, I would then give a little lesson.

"Very good, Meg. A kpiq is a wonderful thing."

I could now spend some class time at the chalkboard, preferably a lot of time, illustrating in great detail any number of objects from my imagination: a pinball machine, a garden gnome, lasagna, tinsel, a forklift. My students loved the tension and anticipation, shouting the Korean words for things they'd guess I was drawing.

Other times, I'd switch to a more student-centred approach.

"Well done, Cabin! Xpligo earns a triple-word score. What do you think it is?"

Up he would go to the chalkboard, and draw a wild guess at something I couldn't make out anyway.

"Yes!" I always said. "Very good, Cabin. That's an xpligo if I ever saw one. Who here has been bitten by a xpligo?"

Because of my approach, when Cabin first speculated I lived in a cabin, I had to agree. My kind of education demanded it.

"Yes, that's where Lion teacher lives. It's my house in Canada."

We shared oohs and ahs, and the picture of my home was passed around for closer inspection. Everybody resumed their chatter, a few of the kids added a chimney, bears, and wilderness to my home, a few kids gave up on me altogether, and the chases I'd interrupted earlier began all over again.

At least my dynamic as a teacher took some shape now. I'd be alright as long as everybody sat still, as long as I held their attention. Serious lessons wouldn't work. In a commotion I'd be at a loss to find anybody or manage my own body among twenty frantic children. How to get by with my employers would be another matter. It's only a few hours a day, I reassured myself. Certainly I could pass for sighted a few hours a day. Besides, I was born and raised in a log cabin. Among my kids, I could move as slowly and strangely as I needed. They would come to know it as Canadian, that's all.

I handed my pen back to the grinning girl.

"Thank you," I said, and realized I didn't know who belonged to the grin. "And what is your name?"

"My name is Shampoo."

"Shampoo?"

Second to the bottom of my list, I found Shampoo, and below her, finishing off the class, I found Conditioner. They were best friends.

For the remainder of that first class, everybody went nuts. Instead of teaching, which is to say making stuff up, I busied myself with orientation, a wary Canadian shuffling about and touching the room into shape. A globe here, a box of pens here, some books there, flashcards in this drawer. Class time would be the easiest task in my new home. The rest of my life and time would be the real work and the real mess.

The move to Pusan had started a couple of months earlier, in the summer of 1996. I was halfway through my graduate degree, and Tracy, unsatisfied with academia, had dropped out. None could believe her bravery. Quitting school? Loan collectors could find you. People with names like Will Powers and Lucy Duty would fill your call display. Although Tracy and I practically lived together, I worried that her leaving the program would give her little reason to stay in Vancouver, a city she'd only moved to for graduate studies. Her family and friends remained back in Saskatoon, not the most hopping place on the planet, but certainly stiff competition for Mr. Magoo and his rainy, minimum-wage city.

One night, over a game of pool with our friend, Reg, both he and Tracy toyed with the idea of teaching overseas. Tracy leaving would be torment, but Reg augmented the threat. The idea of my closest friends jet-setting for jobs without me was too much. I might as well live in some remote log cabin as stay in Vancouver.

I considered my options. I could follow them, earn a salary, and see a part of the world I knew nothing about, or I could stay in lonesome Vancouver and continue my studies, its reading load crippling me daily with headaches and eye-strain. At the time I was in a graduate seminar about V. S. Naipaul and postcolonial literary theory. Yee-haw, you bet. That afternoon four students had debated for two hours whether we had the right to discuss Naipaul's books. As fate

would have it, I'd sat too far from the window to throw myself
out. South Korea with Tracy looked great. It was V. S.
Naipaul's fault, too. I didn't want to read anything by a guy
who said only a blind man could write a book as unreadable
as *Finnegans Wake*. Better things could be done with my failing eyesight. Following Tracy to the other side of the world
seemed like a good start.

The three of us found a recruiter in Vancouver. Mr. Kim
would arrange jobs, airfare, and accommodations. Reg
quickly took a position in Seoul, while Tracy and I waited for
an opening for two instructors at one school. When the jobs
in Pusan appeared, our recruiter phoned with the news and
asked for our documents to fax first thing in the morning. He
needed a copy of our undergraduate degrees and a photograph. A coffee shop meeting was arranged.

We'd only spoken to Mr. Kim over the phone, so he
needed one more bit of information from me.

"How will I recognize the two of you?" he asked.

"Tracy has long brown hair," I said, then realized that
wasn't going to help. "I have a shaved head. I also carry a
white cane because of my eyes."

"A white cane?" he said.

"Didn't I mention it?"

"No." Mr. Kim was stunned. "You're blind?" he asked.

"Uh, somewhat. Not totally. I can still see. Sort of."

I waited for him to say something, but a tense pause built
between us. My only hope was to play down his misgivings.

"It's no big thing. By day you probably can't tell, not really.
I move a bit slow, and I sometimes use my cane just in case."

"Just in case? I don't understand. So you can see?" He was as confused as anybody would be.

"Yes, I can see. A bit. Enough, I mean. It's like looking through a little tunnel in one eye. Around that it's like wavy water, and just waves all through the other one."

"Hmmm." He sounded as if he'd put something together only to find an extra part left over. "This may be a problem, yes? How will you teach?"

Two jobs at one school, Mr. Kim had insisted, don't happen often. I didn't want to blow our chance.

"No, don't worry, I can teach," I said, although I'd never considered how. "I can read and all that. Most people don't even know I'm blind. Going blind, I mean."

"Well, hmmm, okay," Mr. Kim said, clearly reluctant. "The school may not like it. The school must look excellent."

"That's fine," I said. "I'll just keep it to myself, then. They don't need to know, okay? They won't be able to tell, I'm sure. Tracy helps me if I need it, but they won't even notice."

He grumbled, tiring of the debate. I could hear, though, that Mr. Kim was worried. If he sent the school a blind teacher, he could lose status and reputation, which meant he could lose business. The airfare provided to us guaranteed that if we were fired for any reason, we could be sent home immediately. Our school would own our work visas, too. We could teach for them and nobody else, so they had to be pleased with our performance. Mr. Kim's job, in part, was to screen us.

The subject changed to Mr. Kim's next concern.

"And you have no hair?" he asked.

"Nope."

He grumbled some more, probably wondering what the hell kind of dud Tracy had hitched herself to.

"Do you have a picture with hair in it?"

"Oh, sure, just slightly older." By slightly older I meant the picture was from high school, but there was no need to crush the man.

"Okay. Just make sure you have copies of your degrees and your pictures with you tomorrow."

Two weeks later Tracy and I stepped out of the Pusan airport and were greeted, according to Tracy's report, by the astonished expressions of our employers, Mr. and Mrs. Yun. We loaded our luggage into their Hyundai and headed for our new home.

"You have eaten?" Mrs. Yun asked, turning to face us in the back seat. Mr. Yun drove.

"Yes," Tracy said, "we ate on the plane, thank you. We're just very tired."

"I think you will eat?" Mrs. Yun asked.

"You think we will eat?" I asked back.

"Okay," said Mrs. Yun. Our new desire to eat cheered her.

Tuning my ear to this idiom took time. Imperatives always came in the form of questions. Off we went to dinner, where more questions began to command us.

On our table a waiter placed bowls of sticky rice and fish soup. I could smell seaweed, cabbage, and garlic. The affirmation I'd truly arrived overseas came with the aroma. The knowledge and meal were both strong, and for a moment, a rare moment in my time with blindness, I was excited by the future.

"You have no hair," Mrs. Yun observed, "but, um, your picture, it is hairy."

"Oh, yes, I cut it off. It's easier this way, and it isn't so ugly."

"I think it is not so ugly with hair," said Mrs. Yun.

Her tone was difficult to decipher. Perhaps she wanted me to grow my hair again, or perhaps she was being complimentary.

The meal now on the table, I probed discreetly for my chopsticks. I reached for a spot where I thought they might be, but Tracy, spying this strange gesture, as if I was about to play a piano, scooped my chopsticks, and jammed them into my hand. Later she said I was close to stabbing my fingers into my dinner.

"I think you will grow hair?" Mrs. Yun continued.

"I will?"

"Good."

Mr. Yun fed clumps of noodles into his mouth. I tried to imitate him but I couldn't pinch one strand with my thin, metal chopsticks, let alone snag a nest of them. Dinner might take me the term of our contract. Without looking up, Mr. Yun further exposed the hair problem.

"In Korea," he said, and rubbed his head with his free hand, "no hair is meaning two things." He paused and looked for the English words. "You are, how you say—" He turned to Mrs. Yun and consulted her in Korean.

"My husband means you are criminal," she said, "a criminal who was in prison. You are free now? You are that or you are angry at government. At the government. You will eat this?"

I could see her pointing, but not the target. Tracy quickly handed me a bowl. "I think it's pumpkin," she said, and tried a little before she set it down with a thump beside my rice. The sound placed the bowl within a pattern, within my memory of the table. Now I could find and return to the spot. "It's wonderful," Tracy added.

Throughout the rest of the meal, she conjured a variety of reasons to hand me things, preempting any of my usual groping. Neither of us could articulate it yet, but Tracy and I sensed the all-consuming position we'd confined her to. Whether or not my blindness would have prevented us from finding jobs or keeping jobs wasn't clear. It didn't matter anymore. Either way, we weren't prepared to test the status of my disability now. We'd come too far, and we had too much to lose—an apartment, the experience, a good salary. Together we would keep blindness from interfering in our prospects, which meant, in this new country, Tracy would watch, catch, guide, cover, deflect, and mediate for me. She would live two lives, hers and mine, at least when we were around the Yuns or around the school. Given their reaction to baldness, what kind of reception could blindness earn? Keeping my eyes out of sight wasn't my job or struggle anymore. It was Tracy's.

After the meal, the four of us stood to leave the otherwise empty restaurant. Tracy took me by the arm, holding herself close to me, as if too much in love to contain herself. Discreetly she guided me to the car this way. I felt, as I would

139

for the next five months, like a wagon. My empty hand craved a cane the way some lips crave the weight of a cigarette.

As we walked to the car, Mrs. Yun turned to look at us. Occasionally Tracy pointed and observed the city, the architecture, window displays, whatever. Doing so, she covertly described things, prefacing with, "Hey, look at the . . ." or "Did you notice that . . ."

"I think you are very much in love?" Mrs. Yun asked.

"Yes," I said, "we're very close."

In our new neighbourhood, our visibility made for trouble we hadn't anticipated. We were the only western expatriates. Statistically, that's as conspicuous as a pair of fuzzy, pink, oversized gloves on the body politic. Tracy and I would walk to the local corner store for noodles and juice, and, all the way, hear hellos shouted from the apartment buildings high above. Without fail, we returned hellos to the sky. Then another hello would come from another direction. As soon as we hit the street, the signals bounced back and forth. I've never felt so welcomed and so witnessed. Our presence was a paradox I'd only read about: we were the immigrants, both anonymous and overexposed.

So, I couldn't use my cane around our neighbourhood. School wasn't the only no-tapping zone. Too many of the local kids were our students. Too many of their parents owned the local shops and barbecue halls we frequented. Word would get back about the weird teacher bumping into poles at night or caning his way around a herd of idle scooters. Mr. Kim's admonition still needled in my ears. The school must look excellent.

Mr. Yun made admiring his school his primary occupation. He was literally everywhere, wandering the streets with his chest puffed out and his hands clasped behind his back, like some haughty, fallen character from a Dickens novel, all pomp and pride. We'd often find him outside, talking to parents or gazing proudly at the school's new sign.

Meanwhile, Mrs. Yun, a shrewd and gifted business-woman, ran the show. She even opened an illegal franchise for three to five year olds on another floor. We knew she hadn't paid for the licence because, when inspectors came around, we were told to lock down the new floor and make all the children sit silently or nap. Warning usually came in advance of an inspection because Mr. Yun saw the franchise reps coming while he either strolled up and down the street or smoked on the corner with the school's bus drivers.

The ubiquity of Mr. Yun caused my other problem. Because we couldn't count on where he was at any given moment, my cane stayed at home, and Tracy stayed on my elbow, even on a short run to the market for squid-flavoured chips. We learned our lesson about Mr. Yun within days. One afternoon, looking for a place to eat, I caned around a corner, Tracy just behind me, and walked smack into the owner of a lunch cart. Mr. Yun was on the other side of the cart, too focused on eating and yakking with people to have noticed my collision.

I collapsed my cane in one fluid move, like a soldier would his rifle. Tracy shoved it in her purse. Arm in arm, as always, we walked around and were greeted by Mr. Yun's surprise.

"I think you are hungry?" he asked.

He held up a long, thin skewer with what looked to me like a brown lump on the end.

"Very good," he said and dipped the lump in some sauce before biting a chunk. "You will eat?"

Before we could answer, Mr. Yun ordered two freshly made lumps. Tracy, a fickle eater, and a salad in a previous life, was wary.

"What is it, Mr. Yun? I can't eat red meat."

Mr. Yun was perplexed, his English extremely limited.

"Beef," Tracy explained. "I cannot eat," she searched for the Korean word, "bulgogi?"

To illustrate her idea of a bad lunch, I made a pair of horns with my fingers and planted them on my forehead. Bull face.

Mr. Yun smiled with recognition. "No, no," he laughed. "Here, for you." He handed me a heavy skewer and clarified my lunch's name. "Feces," he said.

I'd heard Shampoo correctly, but I didn't want to hear feces or hold it on a skewer. It couldn't be true, I told myself, and I didn't want to be one of those narrow-minded tourists who'd believe something like a thriving, fecal cuisine was a Pusan favourite. But my paranoia was well lubricated. It's a common state of mind when you can't see.

Together, language and sight, unable to clarify for me, made ample room for distaste and fear. Without the native tongue and without the ability to see Korea for myself, I was already regressing into a gullible kid, one who could believe anything, especially if it was brown and unidentifiable and destined for my mouth.

"Feces?" I checked.

"Yes," Mr. Yun beamed. "Good feces."

Tracy stifled a laugh, then whispered in my ear, "Don't be a total idiot. He's saying fishes. You missed the swimming-hand gesture."

In guarding my blindness, I was habituating daily to a character I didn't much like. Pretending to be sighted, or passing for sighted, demands a blind person establish a functional degree of self-loathing and fretfulness. With a generous skewer of fish in hand, my duplicity suddenly occurred to me for what it was—a sour and potentially chronic state of mind, one in which I believed everything and everybody could get me if I didn't pass for sighted.

Even Mr. Yun did his best to meet somewhere between us, stretching his English and offering me what he could of his home. I, on the other hand, was doing little to meet him or anybody at the school. Assuming the worst, acting reserved, withdrawn, dubious, and indifferent—these were my defences for my secret. In my mind, being closed would keep me from being dismissed, sent from a place I was more or less avoiding. The only person dishing out shit around here was me. It left a bad taste.

For longer than I care to recall, that lunch with Mr. Yun was the last time I took my cane anywhere in our neighbourhood. It may have also been the last time I heard Tracy laugh in South Korea.

Tracy's burden with my blindness was the same every day, but over weeks and months, without variation or relief, the strain accumulated. I couldn't leave the apartment, not alone, not without endangering myself on the streets. Instead, I made it my job to pace or sleep my free time away, feeling stifled, cramped, and sorry for myself. When Tracy did guide me out, our time became another kind of entrapment, me perpetually slung on her arm like a bag. I felt the weight of it, and she felt it even more.

What she experienced, for the first time, was her own independence disappearing, overtaken by my visual needs and depression. Like the neighbouring hillside, the one riddled with landmines, my independence here was both off-limits and a historical artifact. But it wasn't simply about walking around. Tracy had to do just about everything for both of us.

Once, at the Nampo-dong market, she let go of my elbow to choose some vegetables. As anybody would, I began to roam, keeping near, but shimmying around crowds of shoppers. I felt the nearby shelves and baskets of goods to discover what they held.

A friend once described to me the single-frame newspaper comic I was about to imitate. In it a storekeeper and his jittery expression are stuck behind the counter. A blind man is about to take his next step into a large pyramid of neatly displayed light bulbs. I saw the comedy in it, but I had to wonder what stupid hardware chain would build a pyramid of light bulbs in the middle of an aisle, in front of the checkout, no less. At the Nampo-dong market I didn't find a tower of light bulbs, lucky for me and the guy in the light bulb department. My shoulder, however, did find the edge of a five-foot column of clear, plastic egg cartons, a dozen white eggs in each.

Within the translucent cartons, both the eggs and the white floor tiles mixed and matched enough to disappear. An empty white aisle. It looked like that, until I heard the display. I clipped it with my shoulder. Plastic creaked and leaned. I wheeled around, saw what hadn't been there before, then caught a bit of a stranger's hand clamping down on top of the eggs. The motion stopped, and I thanked my savior in equally unsteady Korean.

Tracy, a few feet away, about to pay for our vegetables, caught the climax of the scene and was on me like a carton on a dozen loose eggs. She was furious.

"Just, just—I don't know. Just don't, okay? Just don't. You almost knocked over the eggs."

Because I see so little, I protect its territory. When somebody, anybody, notes a calamity I've barely sidestepped, but one I'm already fully aware of, I burn. This was one of those moments.

"I know I hit the eggs. You don't have to tell me that. I'm not an idiot. I know what I did. And don't blame me. I didn't see them. Who the hell leaves eggs in the middle of the aisle, anyway?"

To defend myself, I hoped to fault others, a tactic my siblings and I perfected on one another when we were kids. It still didn't work.

"What are you talking about?" Tracy said. "The world is not conceived and designed just for you. That includes South Korea."

"But eggs should be refrigerated. Who expects eggs when—"

"It's not about the eggs or what you expect."

"Yes, it is."

"No, it isn't!"

"Well, what am I supposed to do without my cane? Just stand here, do nothing because I can't be certain I'll walk into a bunch of eggs? It's stupid. All I can do is, I don't know, *expect.* I have to expect my way around."

Tracy was exasperated. She told me to drop it, but I've never been good at letting anything go, be it sight or arguments.

"No, seriously," I continued, "what am I supposed to do? Nothing? Wait for you all the time? I might as well stay home for the rest of the year. If I bump into stuff, you're not responsible, so just let me."

"Why would I do that? You want me to let you knock things over while I watch? Okay, fine. But that's really stupid, not where the eggs are kept."

"But I need you to—"

"I don't want to talk about this here," she said. "Just let it go."

"But I think—"

"Just let—it—go."

I could hear the approaching bind, so I shut up. If I pushed the point, she would want to walk away, but couldn't, or wouldn't. She never had, and I didn't want to drive her to it now. I could be stubborn and prodding when we bickered, but Tracy, for some reason, never left me helpless, never used my eyes to put some sting in her point. We could have been in a heated exchange on our way out of the apartment, over something small but symbolic. If at that moment I groped about for my jacket and couldn't find it, Tracy would hand it to me while the argument carried on. She didn't want to talk about our problems now, so I let it go and let us go home.

Within a couple of months, we found ourselves in the same angry scenes more and more often. Always having me on her arm, Tracy's own feeling of entrapment soon overwhelmed her signature patience and generosity. We were, officially, too close.

In the beginning our office-apartment was unfurnished, and we were too broke to buy anything beyond a few essentials: propane tanks for the hotplate, towels, bedding and whatnot. The previous teachers had left pots and pans, a kitchen table, a couple of chairs and a sleeping mat, but that's about it. Tracy, alone, over a few months, filled in the rest.

Some evenings she cruised the alleys and sidewalks for discarded furniture or wooden crates, anything we could use for tables and chairs and shelves. The supply was out there, but our means were limited: I couldn't help. Tracy needed both hands to carry things, and in no way could I walk on my own in the dark. When she combed the alleys, she always returned with something for our apartment, including more frustration. One night she found a couch. Another capable body was needed. Instead of coming home for help, she stopped at the school in search of a willing teacher. What excuse she gave for me, I don't know. It must have been humiliating, though, asking a colleague to help salvage trash on my behalf. Indeed we were too close, on top of one another all the time. But when she needed me, somehow I wasn't there, either.

Her new life may have been harder than anything I've had to reconcile. Despite love, Tracy was finding her compassion exhausting. To carry blindness, we were learning a sighted partner must give up some of her own ability to see and the life it makes, as she'd come to know it. That was a sacrifice our companionship demanded, and one I will always regret for her. Neither of us could accept the cost. It took our isolation in another culture, without others to speak to, and the secrecy of my condition, all these exaggerations, to reveal blindness as we'd never known it before: as much hers as mine.

After five months our problems found little voice. We did our best to keep the issues down, way, way down, but their expression eventually found a vocabulary: sex. It disappeared. In retrospect, it couldn't have survived. We both taught children and then, when Tracy arrived home, she tended to me, aided me, guided me, and watched my self-imposed helplessness. I blurred into one of her kids, and she morphed into a full-time mother. The last thing she wanted at the end of the day was to be physically close. Our mattress on the floor became the single place she could find space for herself. Meanwhile, I lay awake, needing to offer something and to feel like a man and a lover, not a little boy or luggage.

The crisis found one other expression, both small and final. One morning I sat on our dirty couch, counting down the minutes until class. For three days I hadn't left the building, which wasn't uncommon. It was my only way to assert independence. Most mornings I walked down the three floors to the school, taught—well, horsed around—then walked back upstairs and stayed in. The Green Boy restaurant delivered food, soup or pizza, albeit pizza with corn, so I had little reason to leave. On this particular morning, Tracy sat cross-legged on the floor blow-drying her hair, neither of us speaking. Then, without cause, from what I could tell, she shut off the dryer and leapt onto the couch, muttering, "Shit, oh, shit, oh . . ." Like a dog alerted to a distant sound, I sat up and scanned.

"What? What's wrong?"

"It's a roach," she said, "a huge, huge roach." She stared somewhere at the floor. "Oh, shit."

If I rummaged around my memory, I bet every girlfriend I've had has at some point leapt from bugs while in my presence. If I could see, I would, too. Not many things make me squeamish. Snakes do. Roaches do, too. Very squeamish.

"Where is it?" I said as I pulled my feet up onto the couch.

Not that I imagined a roach beside my bare feet. I imagined all of them. Why even have a singular form? Never a roach, always roaches. Tracy didn't answer me, so I pressed.

"C'mon, where is it?"

Maybe she was now and forever paralysed on the couch, staring at one of a thousand belt-buckle-sized bugs. Our new roommates. We slept on the floor. I was thinking about that, as I'm sure Tracy was, if she wasn't already designing in her mind some sort of hammock system we could sling from the ceiling.

She muttered one more "Oh, shit," and in it I heard a tone I didn't recognize, nor wanted to recognize. It was defeat, a pure, flat surrender. That was it. She'd had enough. Of everything.

"Tell me where it is," I insisted.

"It's on the floor, but don't bother—"

"Where on the floor?"

She was impatient. "Just, I don't know, on the floor. On the floor, over there."

"Where's there?"

"Where I was!"

"Okay, okay. How am I supposed to know? Is it near the low table?"

"No," she sighed, "near the chair."

I didn't need antennae to get the signal. Tracy was trying to figure out what to do next, while I was, like the roach, bugging her.

"I'll get it," I said.

The prospect of roach hunting didn't thrill me, but I needed to help, anything to lift Tracy up. It was just a bug, that's all. I didn't want it to become anything more than that. I didn't want a symbol, be it for blindness, for my failure to help, for anything. Kill it while it's still a bug and get rid of whatever Tracy was feeling.

She began to say something, telling me not to move, but I was off the couch and shuffling towards an idea of where the roach might be.

"Is it around here?" I whispered. I think I didn't want it to hear my plan.

Tracy's voice was full and steely. "No, it's gone. I said 'don't move' and now it's run somewhere." I stared hard at the floor, as if she might be wrong. "Thanks," she added.

"Holster the sarcasm. I'm trying to help. Where'd it go?"

"It's gone under the book-crates, but just don't, okay? Just forget it."

"No, I can do it."

"No," she said, "no, you can't."

She'd never said that to me before, and it was more than either of us wanted to hear. It was, in a word, true. She turned the blow-dryer back on and resumed getting ready for work. I gave up and sat back down on the couch.

I can't say I was disappointed that Tracy thought I couldn't kill a bug in our house. Disappointment is too small. I was emasculated, enraged at her, at the roach, at blindness, at fast-moving children, at our skuzzy home, at Mr. Yun and his inability to sit at his desk, at my distrust in Korea, at unrefrigerated eggs, at the weight of couches, at everything, including my own complicity. Why couldn't I just be a blind person, here or at home? I didn't know how to let go of my sight, in a way Tracy could live with. In a way I could live with.

We sat on the couch and stared at the crates where the roach lived. It was probably multiplying already, the way symbols do. Like me, it could stay home in the dark indefinitely. It could have, but it didn't. A few minutes passed, and it crawled out again. This time I spotted it. The little body fit just inside my sliver of sight, filling my good eye with black and gloss. I picked a book up from the coffee table and tried to come down with one quick move.

"It's not there," Tracy said.

Normally she would've found this funny, me killing the floor. But she sounded tired. My attempts to do as the sighted

do are sometimes laughable, but only so long as we're not trying to accomplish anything.

"Where is it, then?"

"Never mind. It doesn't matter. You won't get it."

Her certainty, and her withdrawal, hurt.

"Well, then, why don't you try," I snapped. "At least I'm
trying."

Tracy shut off the blow-dryer again. "I'm tired of trying,"
she said and meant all of it. Whatever she'd found in herself,
I couldn't catch or contain. Her blur stood up and walked
away, then shut the bedroom door between us.

Mrs. Yun had been organizing a large-scale musical, an
English extravaganza to be performed by all the students. We
were slotted to help with rehearsal that morning. The cast's
pronunciation of lines and songs from *Willy Wonka and the
Chocolate Factory* needed serious coaching. I feigned enthusiasm, but I didn't need six hours of know-it-all Oompa
Loompas telling me what sort of lesson I should learn from a
kid who chews too much gum or a kid who watches too
much TV. At least their deviances earned novel transforma-
tions—a girl who becomes a blueberry, a boy who shrinks to
the size of a glue stick. Nobody, not even an Oompa Loompa,
had warned me what would happen to a blind guy who
refuses to close his eyes.

I walked into the rehearsal room with Tracy's shadowy figure just ahead of me, the shape offering a little guidance. My
favourite student, Little John, the smallest, most animated
boy in Apple Class, jumped between us and greeted his
teacher, the Lion King. Lots of other kids picked on Little

John, a name I gave him because the plainer "John" was already taken by a dour Christian boy. Little John remembered the character from Robin Hood and was happy I saw it in him. Most mornings he ran to greet me before any of the others.

Bounding in front of me, waist high, he looked up and shouted, "Good morning, Lion King!" Overcome with enthusiasm, he seized my nuts in one hand and gave them a nasty rattle, shaking hello. To my surprise, they were still there.

I had to do something. Since Pusan was going down fast, I decided I'd rather lose my job than lose Tracy. By the end of the day, I was determined to out myself with my cane. It may have been too late, but we needed to see if any light could get in.

As a first act, I told Tracy I would be going out the next day on my own, to give her some time to herself. Our friend Reg was scheduled to arrive from Seoul by train in the afternoon. It was our day off.

"You do whatever you like," I said. "I'll get Reg, and we'll be here in time for us all to grab dinner somewhere."

Tracy was both surprised and skeptical. "How? You can't," she said, apparently too comfortable with the phrase. "How will you find anything?"

"I'll use my cane. I know which subway stop it is. I'll find Reg, no problem. Don't worry."

"What, you're going to use your cane now?"

"I think I'd better, don't you?"

"What about the Yuns?"

"I don't know. We'll see."

Tracy didn't contest the idea. She shared, although unspoken, my sense that we didn't have much to lose. If my blindness meant as much as Mr. Kim led us to think, so be it. We'd carry on, find other work, or go home. It wasn't worth it anymore.

The next morning I stepped out of the apartment and down the stairs, tapping the edge of each with my cane. It felt, to understate the point, magnificent. If I ever have my eyes replaced with working models, I bet my first step out of the hospital will feel as good as those first steps with my cane. I could see again. Each tap made definition and let me plod into some rickety kind of freedom. As I rounded the final landing and began to descend the final flight, Mr. Yun strolled through the entrance and climbed the stairs towards me.

"Good morning," he said. "What did you eat?"

Since our day at the lunch cart, Mr. Yun obsessed over our daily menu.

"Kal-gook-su," I said. My pronunciation sucked, but he got the gist of the word I was after. He clapped his hands and laughed, pleased by my effort. We stood on the stairs beside each other, and I leaned somewhat on my cane, waiting.

"What this is?" he asked and plucked the cane lightly, like a stand-up bass.

"It's a stick," I said and tapped it against the stair.

"Ahhhhhh. A stick."

"Yes, a stick."

"Why stick?"

It may not have been the correct answer, but I gave him what I thought was the truth.

"Well, mobility can be a problem, but my stick keeps me in gainful employment."

"A stick is for—?" He tried to repeat some of the phrase but couldn't manage all the syllables.

"Gainful employment," I repeated.

My Scrabble lessons, of all sources, had taught me something of value. I was going to put it to use. If I couldn't hide my cane, I'd try to hide it from reference. If we can't talk about it, we can't talk about it. Tracy and I knew that all too well.

"Ahhhh," he said, after some tutoring, "a stick for gain-ful-em-ploy-ment."

"Very good pronunciation."

"Thank you," he said. "And gainful employment is?"

"It's hard to explain. Difficult." I exaggerated my lean on the cane and motioned to the general scene of us chatting on the landing. "Gainful employment."

"Aaaaah," he said.

"Okay?"

"Okay," Mr. Yun agreed, happy with his new phrase. With that, he said good morning and climbed the stairs.

Tracy and I never saw another blind person in Pusan. If we did, their canes may have differed from mine, or maybe the lack of blindness in the public eye, because of cultural and political pressures, made the use and meaning of a white cane ambiguous for some, such as Mr. Yun. Either way, he accepted my gainful employment and never expressed any interest in the subject again. English was never something he had much interest for in the first place. For the final few weeks that Tracy and I lived in the school and saw the Yuns, I carried my cane and never used its name. Sometimes I carried it in a bundle under my arm, just in case I needed it, and sometimes I walked with it as I did at home, testing the way, casually, with my idiosyncratic style. Back then I didn't swing it much. I tested my path, stabbing down, like a gondolier might test water for depth. Sometimes I used it like a walking stick. Maybe that image of me and my cane never said "blind man" to the Yuns or the other teachers. Perhaps it was a matter of politeness and privacy. Nobody said much about it either way, as if they couldn't see the blindness I'd been hiding after all.

Whatever the truth is, I changed my ways, and although I wore my retinas on my sleeve, when I picked up Reg at the train station, nobody seemed to see me there, either.

Chuffed by my success with Mr. Yun and the promise that things around home might change for the better, I left the school, caned to the subway stop, and made my way to the train station. Despite the thick crowds of people, all of us sandwiched shoulder to shoulder in the subway car, I felt as if I'd inherited an empty city. I was on my own, without my hand on Tracy's elbow. All the way I hummed a Charlie Feathers tune in honour of the occasion. *Leave me one hand loose, and I'll be satisfied . . .*

Emerging from the subway, I walked out onto a public square, across the street from the train depot. As I stepped out, I met Neil, a guy from Oregon who also taught English at another school, one of the few foreigners we'd befriended. The square was crowded with people, although nobody seemed to be moving. Neil and I exchanged greetings. He knew about my blindness but didn't really understand or believe it until he saw me now with a cane. His greeting had a trace of surprise in it.

"What's going on in the square?" I asked.

"You didn't hear about this? It's a protest. There're police and students everywhere."

"What's the cause?"

"Environmental stuff. One of the rivers is being polluted upstream. A smelter or something, I think."

I listened to the protest but couldn't hear anything I recognized as protesting.

"Is it finished?" I asked.

Neil looked around for me. "No, I don't think so. A lot of them are still sitting."

"So it's like a sit-in?"

"Kind of. Students do that here, and a lot of them shave their heads in solidarity."

I felt the breeze on my scalp. Neil noticed what he'd just said.

"Hey!" he chirped. "You fit right in. Better steer clear of the cops."

I looked over Neil's shoulder at the crowd and tried to see the layout of things, where all the bald protesters might end and where a line of cops might begin. Neil realized, again, the implication of what he'd said.

"Do you need me to help you find your way around?"

I did, but I didn't want to give up my first day on my own. It was too sweet, too important to hand back now.

"No, I'll be fine. I'll see you later."

Into the throng of mostly seated people, I tapped my way and, banging loudly, hoped to draw enough attention to my cane that people might move out of the way. I didn't know how, otherwise, to say, I'm blind and I need to get through your protest. As I passed, a few hands tugged at my pant leg, suggesting I sit back down. To those people I shrugged, as if to say, I'm bald every day, so I'm not here to sit with you, although I probably would if I had time, thanks. Few moved. My cane wasn't doing its most expressive job.

On the other side of the square I could see what I guessed were the doors to the train station. I lost the image now and again as I walked, so it took me a long time to get there, stopping occasionally to correct my course and recover lost ground. By the time I arrived at the steps leading to the doors, I'd carved a large zigzag through the protesters. My strange route, I guess, alerted the cops to my presence. They couldn't figure out what I was doing, where I was going, or why. To them I was the odd man out—white, wandering and headed towards them, with a stick and a protester's haircut.

I began to climb the handful of depot stairs when one of the cops blocked my way. He yelled at me, perhaps asking questions, and waited impatiently for answers in between. Clearly he took me for a protester, but I wanted him to see me as a blind man, not a dissident man with a stick. Any worry I had that my cane would cause a problem disappeared when the cop walked away, taking my gainful employment with him.

"No!" I shouted, "I'm blind. I don't see!" My cane was gone and I was paralysed on the stairs.

Had I been near our apartment, it might not have been such a big deal. Without a cane I could make my way around most of the school and, if pressed and in daylight, maybe a bit of our neighbourhood, but only because I'd memorized the routes and the number of steps before turning into the grocery store or turning into Apple Class. I didn't know how many steps to take into the train station or how many to take in pursuit of my confiscated cane.

The only thing that could travel was my voice. I yelled in the direction the cop had walked. I thought I could still see him nearby, standing with other cops and probably disarming my lethal mobility aid. I yelled a bit more, looked around at the indifferent crowd, then gave up. Maybe, I thought, Reg would step out and find me after waiting in the station. If not, eventually he'd phone Tracy, and she would come. I'd be obvious to rescue, stranded on the desert island of the busy front steps, immobile, caneless, and impatient to move.

But it never came to that. Another cop approached me and returned my cane. He said something, his tone quiet and apologetic. Twice in one day I'd taken my cane back. When I tapped the edge of the stair, my world at arm's length lit up all over again. I felt the light I'd carried from Vancouver to Pusan and almost lost.

I wish I could say my cane fixed our time in Korea. I was blind again, a strange salvation, but that didn't mean I'd arrived in the movie version of my life. For its happy ending, Tracy and I would've sat around the kitchen table and laughed at old torments and misadventures, confident all was put to rest. We'd liberated Excalibur and brought it home, my cane. In the final scene, Tracy and I might drink tea at our table, smiling and talking with animation. The camera lens would dilate, bringing into the frame the old apartment teeming with cockroaches, our roommates, which, although familiar, seemed to be new, cute, and adorable, a satire of themselves. Just bugs. Our bugs. I'd like to say my cane was enough to conjure an image like that, but it wasn't. A final scene is the stuff of Hollywood and heroes with superpowers. My cane couldn't heal damage done, nor could it reset broken bonds between Tracy and me. It made our final few weeks easier, but mostly it gave Tracy enough distance and independence to remember herself apart from us. That's what she wanted and needed more of. Whether or not I would remain in the picture wasn't something either of us could see.

On my last teaching day, Apple Class spent the hour playing hangman. Cabin chose a word, and I helped him find its spelling in the dictionary. Under his sketch of the gallows he scored a blank space for each letter. Game on. The Megs and Kevins and Batmans shouted words and letters and flipped through their dictionaries. Most of them guessed the oddities, x and q and j, hoping, I suppose, they weren't as rare as they really are. Exotic letters. The hangman was well defined and on his way to the other side, but Cabin carried on, adding details with every incorrect guess. A bald man with glasses and two earrings came into focus. The correct word was "lion." With their hysteria and applause, Apple Class declared my effigy to be the finest gag ever executed. That's how we said goodbye to him, together.

Missing

The moment Tracy and I returned from Pusan, we set out to rediscover our affections and repair our strained bond the only way possible. We separated. Within days of landing in Vancouver, Tracy booked a flight to Saskatchewan. She wanted to see her family. "A couple of weeks," she said. "I just need a couple of weeks."

Four weeks later, I flew to the prairies for a visit, hoping to size up the situation. I needed to find where Tracy's head and heart were at. Both were staying put in Saskatchewan. "Maybe another month," she said, truly uncertain where she wanted to be or what she wanted to do, other than not be in Vancouver with me.

I waited some more, but when an email of hers mentioned a job in a clothing store, I knew I had to evaluate my own direction. I'd lived for the past month in a basement suite roughly the size of my left lung. Take a deep breath, and my subterranean digs emptied of oxygen. And mildew spores. Cash was running low, so I'd applied for a job as an administrative assistant for a nonprofit arts group. Without question, my organizational skills were as sharp as my vision, and I had no office experience to speak of. Luckily for me, none of this surfaced during the interview.

"Ryan, pretend it's a rough morning for a sec. Handle this situation for me. When you arrive at work to open the arts resource centre, several people are already at the door. Two clients want immediate help with grant applications—you know those artists, they just can't wait!—and a third wants to use our library, which isn't open till noon. Entering the office, you hear the phone is ringing and see the message light is blinking. The fax machine looks jammed again, and we're expecting an important document. Among the people waiting is a courier with a package you need to sign for. Think about it, though. The lights haven't been turned on yet, and the sign put out front. The alarm needs the code within a minute, too. So, wow, rough morning. I'd like to know what you'd do first."

"First I'd tell everybody how weird this is. I'm in the same test situation from my job interview. What are the chances?"

I started the next day.

I'm still surprised how easily offices fall apart. Within a month, what hadn't emerged during the interview began to show. My filing system, for one thing, exhibited terminal signs of stress. My system involved three piles of paper: the first for "Things That Need Attention," the second for "Things That Also Need Attention," and the third for "Things That Probably Matter But I Don't Know What To Do With." The third pile towered. Throughout my days I accomplished close to nil, despite putting in a solid eight hours. My ability to read print and find documents in filing cabinets was so slow that it pained even me. The only positive was that I always appeared to be reading or looking for files. I was busy, just not productive. You'd think I typed a lot, too, but it was usually the same page, sometimes several times over, if I couldn't find the white out. Not that I looked hard.

Even though I accomplished little, my eyes and brain ached by five o'clock, unable to keep up with the visual demands of a day. I didn't fit, couldn't do what was asked of me, and didn't want to. Clearly I wasn't trying to make things better for myself, just using my old tactics of denial and avoidance. I wasn't really working or living. I was waiting for Tracy to come home. When she took the job in Saskatchewan, though, I realized that my filing system would collapse, perhaps even kill me, before Tracy would return and resume her old role. It was time to do things for myself, for the first time in a long time. I needed to find my own pace and forget the pace of a life lived at the end of another person's elbow.

To start, I quit my job and re-enrolled at Simon Fraser University, ready to complete my graduate degree. That was where I belonged. I even took a job there, as a teaching assistant. Now I always used my cane, was up front with my professors and students that I was mostly blind, and asserted that it might take me a little longer to read assigned books or to grade papers. Accommodations were made. Nobody flinched, and nobody fired me or threatened deportation. I encouraged myself, willfully, into living within my abilities and my body. I began to assert the need for help, but only when I really needed help. It felt good. Blindness proved easier to manage when I wasn't worrying about its burden on Tracy.

Maybe she understood that from my emails. I can still remember all the work I put into those few lines a day, sentences clotted with overwrought attempts at charm. I wanted them to register how relaxed, adjusted, hopeful, motivated, and satisfied I felt, excepting her absence. Maybe all that was enough to remind her of the young man I'd been before my self-imposed apathy and helplessness. Only she knows. Whatever magic transpired, one day, nearly half a year after we first landed back in Vancouver, Tracy appeared on my doorstep, a surprise, suitcases in hand.

We took our time. She would find her own apartment, and we'd give things another try, close but apart, independent and bound. Not too this, not too that. The Goldilocks theory of commitment. If I could bottle and sell whatever time and method resurrected us, I'd have my own infomercial. In the summer of 1998 I graduated and, after a job interview conducted with my fly down and my blindness, well, out in the open, Capilano College hired me and secured computer technology to help me with reading and teaching. I've remained there, grateful and content, ever since. What's more, Tracy and I found a nice apartment with old wooden floors and cherry trees out front. We moved back in together. We may have had a few remaining ghosts, but we had space to spare and plenty of storage.

The morning of May 12, 1999, I sat in my office, with a stack of unmarked essays on my desk. For me, procrastination always begins with voice mail. I decided to check the messages at home.

Two new messages. Both were marked urgent, so I felt vindicated in having decided to waste time. When I pressed the button, both messages replayed my father's voice in my ear. His tone was terse, flat, yet somehow alarmed. Both messages shared the identical phrasing, too. "Ryan, it's Dad. Call my cell right away." No goofy "Yello," instead of "hello," or "B-bye now," as he always says. Something was off. I called him back and tried not to sound a little worried.

"Hi, Dad. What's going on?" He didn't answer, so my worry grew. "Dad? You there?"

Instead of words, his voice whimpered under his breath. It was gutshot. A pained and quiet sound. A thin, bleeding moan I'd never heard before.

"What happened," I barked.

He began to weep quietly, then more of that moan. He couldn't answer, so without missing a beat, I jumped ahead and cut to the worst bone. "Who?" I said. Just, "*Who*?"

The phone went quiet. I couldn't tell if he was still there but carried on anyway. "Who, Dad? Who? Is it Ma?"

The cell phone rustled in my ear, the sound of it changing hands, then I heard a new voice, a woman's. She said, "Here, Miles, let me talk to him."

"Ma?"

"Ryan?"

"What's—"

"Ryan, it's Auntie Angie. I'm—I'm so—"

"Where's my mother, Angie?" I felt cornered and disoriented, as if pushed into a cave. My eyes grew starry and buzzed with panic. "What happened, Angie?"

"I'm so sorry, Ryan. It's, it's Rory," she said.

My body flooded with relief. This wasn't about my mother—it was about somebody else. Then, almost immediately, my little brother's name registered, and my relief hardened into an icy guilt. Angie continued to talk. She delivered the news as straight and clear as she could, as if teaching a child something new and difficult to understand.

"Ryan, listen to me. Rory took some pills last night," she began. She spoke slowly. "We don't know much more at this point, but I'm here at the hospital with your parents, okay? Everybody did everything they could. He's gone, hon. I'm so sorry, but he's gone."

"Gone?"

Something heavy arrived. Comprehension, its freefall, then a kind of pain that knocks you away from words. Your mind moves far from your body. You don't know if you are alive anymore, you are so numb, so empty, so blown.

"Rory? But, but he can't . . ." I searched for an argument, the one to cheat death with. I couldn't find it.

"I'm so sorry, hon."

"Is there a note?"

"Can you leave work, Ry? Your parents need you, hon. Come to Langley Memorial Hospital. Everybody's here. Your mom, dad, Mykol, and Erin are all here."

The list of names nauseated me. Already Rory was disappearing. He was at the hospital, too, yet not there, among my family's names. I'd recited that list the same way all my life: Mom, Dad, Rory, Mykol, Erin. A name was missing. The new order sounded alien and its expression empty. This wasn't my family.

"But I don't know how to get there," I said, "We don't have a car."

"Can you get a taxi?"

"Did he leave a note?"

"No, hon. There's no note."

"But Tracy's at work."

"Pick her up on the way, okay?"

"Who's there, Angie?"

"Listen to me, Ry. Call a taxi, then pick Tracy up at work, then come to the hospital. Okay? I'll wait for you out front."

"But I don't have any money. I can't take a taxi."

Trauma dreams its own logic. Mine believed, truly, that if I couldn't go to the hospital, Rory couldn't be there. Angie and I carried on this way, trying to sort through my shock, to get me in a cab. When I hung up the phone, I walked across the hall to a colleague's office. Maria, a good friend, stood in front of her bookshelf, looking for something. She said hi and sounded like a smile as I shuffled into her office. I didn't know what to do or how to begin. Angie's instructions were gone. I aimed for Maria's blur, wrapped my arms around it, and said, "My brother just killed himself. Can somebody help me go home?"

Maria and another colleague, Sharon, drove me to my apartment. We walked together to the car, my friends on either side, each holding an arm, guiding and hugging me at once. Soon I was in a taxi. From our apartment I'd called Tracy at work and told her what happened, imitating Angie's calm as best I could. Neither of us cried or said much in the cab on the way to the hospital. We held hands, and I fought the urge to grip Tracy's, though I felt that if I didn't, I'd blow out the open window. "I'll be okay, I'm going to be alright," I repeated. It felt like a test, to see, each time, if the phrase could ever be true.

I wish I could capture all of Rory's character, give the right anecdotes that might illustrate who my little brother was. I struggle, though. It's not for lack of memory, either. I just don't know how to describe him anymore. If you asked me the day before he died, I'd tell you what I like to recall. He's one of those few people I saw when I could see full and well. But everything is different now. Despite the same stories, he becomes a different person than the one I remember. It's frustrating, how his death interprets our memories of him.

Many people, family friends, even Rory's old school chums, probably can't help themselves. They look at his life through the lens of his overdose. Now, when I say Rory is the funniest person I've ever known, it's still true, but his death draws implications. His overdose wants to explain all of him. It can't, and shouldn't. I learned that first at his funeral. Many reminisced with me and agreed that, yes, he was terribly, terribly funny. It appears Rory's humour staved off a kind of despair I'll never have a name for. Maybe it's true, but it saddens the memory of his wit. More importantly, I don't care. I still remember him as the funniest person I've ever known, not the funniest person coping with depression. The question remains with me, how do you describe the dead as they lived? It's similar to the way blindness can own my life, too. Boy, that Ryan sure is one ambitious workaholic, eh? Yeah, seems he won't let that blindness thing slow him down. Truth is, I'm a generic workaholic. Even I struggle not to make my eyes the overwhelming logic of who I've become. Memories and understanding always gravitate to these black holes in our lives. What needs to be said, though, is that Rory's death does not understand much about who he was. Something, but not much. The day he died was only one out of the twenty-one years that made him the person I knew. That's important to me.

I will remember him as theatrical and short, eager to please, a little boy with either a grin on his face or an expression full of flat withdrawal. I will remember how, as a young man, his shape lumbered across the kitchen and hunched its shoulders, strong and thick-bodied, with our father's barrel-chest. I will remember a fist the size of the dent in my parents' refrigerator. He was lonesome and loyal to whoever would have him, explosive only with those who could cope. Bipolar, but misdiagnosed for years. I will remember when Dad was barbecuing, and Rory grabbed him in a slow dance, cooing, "Oh, Miles, oh, Miles." I will remember the time, long after I'd taken up a white cane, Rory let me steer his car while he worked the pedals, just as I'd let him steer when he was a kid. Rory was moral and shocked by injustice. He couldn't understand why Dad sold my car without warning buyers about the oil leak. I will remember the feeling of the thorns tattooed on his inner arm. He always sided with the forgotten and the marginal kids at school. Called my 110-pound sister Fatty, and called me The Gimp. We loved it, but never found the right name for him. So impulsive and so undisciplined. If he was at home, alone, he turned all the lights on. I will remember him planting tomatoes with my grandmother every spring. He bought the heaviest cigarettes and the filterless brands. Impersonated everybody to perfect caricature. Was restless but left town only once. I will remember his bedroom door, open when he slept, and a light on in the corner. When we weren't laughing, he was at war with himself, so we laughed a lot.

To this day it's unclear what happened. We're only left with speculation, which is more brutal than facts. My parents live in a circle of hell where they bear the punishment for all the unanswered questions, all the what-ifs, and nothing, no amount of therapy, time, or advice to "move on," can free them. The sketch of my brother above may suggest that the war with manic depression got the better of him one day, but none of us are so sure.

The morning Rory died, my mother was at Langley's police detachment, where she had started working years ago as a cell matron and quickly moved up in responsibility, soon dispatching 911 calls and now supervising dispatchers in the radio room. She always knew what was going on. You could ask her at any given moment where any of her officers were and why. Without looking at her log, she could tell you. Among her other gifts is foresight. She could anticipate the need for backup and dispatch it before she was asked. At times, she even insisted on such precautions, putting safety ahead of any other priorities. Although she wasn't dispatching anymore, mostly training her younger crew, Ma's desk had a computer screen that showed all incoming emergencies. The morning Rory died, she looked at her screen and saw a call for assistance. It referred to an unresponsive twenty-one-year-old male. The address was Rory's apartment.

Rory lived at the time with a new girlfriend, a woman I'll call Robin. He'd met Robin only weeks earlier and had separated only weeks before that from Paula, his girlfriend of many years and the mother of their one-year-old son, Gavin. Rory's moods and impulsiveness had driven him away from his young family. He'd voluntarily moved back home with my parents to ensure that Gavin and Paula would have a more stable environment. Rory saw his son every day and never raised his voice or lost patience. It wasn't easy, though. He worked hard not to let his black dog loose on anybody that couldn't understand or forgive him. That included his wee son, whom Rory loved most in the world.

Robin was the sister of my brother Mykol's girlfriend, but we'd never met Robin before. She'd lived for years as a heroin addict, marginal even to her own family. Recently she'd emerged from rehab and had moved back to Langley to live with her sister and Mykol. The idea was to get away from her old life on the streets of Vancouver. Rory took to her immediately. Both were people trying to change themselves, and both were lonely and struggling.

My mother's foresight wasn't limited to her work. "You know, Ror, maybe you and Robin should slow down a bit," she'd say, among other things. But Rory, unlike the officers Ma dispatched, didn't listen. He was also twenty-one, not a child anymore, and thoroughly bullheaded, like me. He moved in with Robin in typical style. On impulse.

One day Robin received an inexplicable gift: unsupervised access to a Langley doctor's office. Her mother, of all people, handed over the keys. Robin's mother cleaned the office at night, except on this one occasion, when she asked her addicted daughter to cover a shift. Robin, fresh from rehab, would be alone for the night in a room full of drugs and prescription pads.

What she found, while cleaning and without any difficulty, were two bottles of pills the doctor had left in a box under his desk, along with many other loose narcotics. The box of pills had belonged to various patients who'd either passed away or recovered from their illnesses. The extra medications had been returned for proper disposal but had never been disposed of, as required. Robin pocketed one bottle of Valium and one bottle of liquid morphine in capsule form. To say she felt tempted would imply an inner debate I can't say Robin knew how to have with herself. She brought the pills home and showed Rory her luck. Bad idea. She didn't know Rory at all. To know him is to suspect, at the very least, that a morphine score on the part of his new girlfriend was not his idea of hitting the jackpot.

Only Robin knows what happened next. Rory was neither a user nor an addict, yet it was her drugs that killed him. Her numerous statements during the investigation recall a different story every time and are riddled with contradictions. According to the police, that should come as no surprise, even if she had nothing to hide. An addict's first instinct is self-preservation. Honesty is too dangerous in that pursuit. The only fact her statements share is this: when Rory learned about the drugs, they fought and fought hard. She claims Rory was furious and told her to return the drugs. I've also heard he tried to take them away, to flush them down the toilet. Another statement says he wrestled away some pills and crushed them in a showy rage. Whatever the manner, we know they fought, and at the end of the day, Robin gave Rory two Valium and told him to go to bed. She said the pills would help cool his jets, while she slept on the couch. The autopsy revealed no Valium in his system, though. She'd given him morphine.

The toxicology report showed an amount roughly equivalent to two pills. It was just enough, just marginally enough for his age and body weight, to shut his system down. According to one of Robin's statements, he went to bed angry, and in the morning, he was snoring heavily. She couldn't wake him, so she left him to sleep some more. The next time she tried to wake him, he wasn't breathing right.

So much doesn't make sense and never will. Why would he take the very drugs he was so angry about? One story says he asked for the Valium, another that she put them in his hand and said, "Here, take these." Did he know what the pills really were? Did she know? Was it a deliberate switch, to get him to try the morphine? Maybe she thought he'd like it and let her keep the pills. Or was it just the most costly mix-up of his life? And then back again: why would he take anything he was that opposed to? Two pills is not a suicide, either. What is it we're left with? Little and nothing. Death. Unreliable accounts and a cruel set of contradictions. We stare into the facts, but nothing takes final shape. Just this sketchiness, just our inferences, our conjectures, the same way I look at the world and navigate through its smear, hoping the errors won't hurt too much.

Within days of Rory's death, Robin's ex-boyfriend, also a junkie, moved into the apartment. My father and sister arrived one afternoon to gather Rory's things. Robin's boyfriend, flopped out on Rory's couch, was playing my brother's Sega games.

Acquiring knowledge is one way my mother grieves. For years she has wrestled in private with her sadness about my eyesight. But that battle, like any of hers, quickly translated itself into practical action. After my diagnosis, she couldn't help me through the process of going blind. I'd moved out too quickly. Instead, because she needed to help, she immersed herself in all the literature and research. To this day she knows more about the science of my retinas than I do. Occasionally, and cautiously, she updates me about clinical trials I would otherwise ignore. We both know my psyche can't afford to place all hope in the remoteness and bureaucracy of scientific progress. A life is not best built around the idea that maybe the cure is near. But my mother is out there, following it on my behalf. The moment a solid breakthrough blips on the radar, I'll get a call.

That's what she does when one of her family is in trouble. She does everything she can to get some control back for those who seem helpless or lost. Hers is a generous will to power, through knowledge. For years she'd done everything she could to help Rory, too. Nutritionists, psychologists, psychiatrists, physicians, even dance lessons to help Rory develop a different relationship to his body and nervous energy. Based on what she knew, she developed her own approach. If he was furious and manic about something, Ma would send him downstairs to write her a letter before they'd talk. Writing gave him clarity and tempered his mood beforehand. And what moods they were. I remember when she quietly dispatched my father, like one of her officers, to disconnect the starter in Rory's car, a necessary tactic before she confronted Rory about something he'd done. Ma didn't want her son taking off at fifty miles an hour, past the elementary school, in a pissed-off rage. "If he bolts," she said, "a run will do him good."

Of course Ma was out the door, chasing after the 911 call, already sharing blame for something she could never have foreseen or prevented. When she arrived at Rory's apartment, she burst through the bedroom door to find paramedics trying to resuscitate her son. A couple of hours earlier she'd phoned the house, and Robin had said he was sleeping, although it was late. It's been six years, and still Ma will be busy with her rose bushes, or scrubbing the day's forks and knives, then prick with black thought. How close she came to insisting Robin wake Rory up. Maybe the difference of those two hours would have made all the difference. Nobody knows. As if anybody could have seen it coming. If foresight and hindsight had their own eyes in our bodies, my mother would have blinded hers by now. I would help her do it, too, just to give her some peace.

By the time Tracy and I arrived at the hospital, everybody except Auntie Angie had left. Nothing more could be gained or hoped for there, so my parents and brother and sister had gone home, to our family house, to—to what? To rage, to pace? Do what? Make dinner? Stare at nothing? What do you do inside the vacuum?

Daily I'm accosted by things that hurt: chairs, half-open doors, sandwich boards, even dogs, the ones I sometimes discover with the tip of my cane. Usually accidents are small, but sometimes they're hefty, landing me in a clinic or the emergency ward. Often I go to work looking like a boxer, bruised and mulched by whatever my face hammers. The bodies of the blind grow more and more conditioned. We rebound from the world, suck up the sting, and push ahead. It seems inevitable in our character to carry on, like the Terminators of this world. I defer to the wisdom of the blues. As my friend Harmonica Slim says, when I'm particularly bruised or gashed, "Well, kid, you ain't good looking, but you're hard to kill."

Maybe that's why, driving home in Angie's car, I promised myself that I could do the same now, carry on for my family. I would take the lead. Let them rest, lose their minds, whatever they needed. I would be one step ahead, thrashing about, clearing the way for them. Arrangements needed to be made: phone calls to family, Rory's friends, Rory's landlord and bank, the coroner. A mountain of pebbles needed moving. Even the tiny but insurmountable stuff had to keep up. Groceries, meals, dishes piling in the sink. Whatever it took, I'd do it or keep things going. But not a tear until I was done. That was the promise I made and kept. It was selfish, too. I needed to know that when my family looked around, they'd see somebody holding it together. I hoped the image, even the illusion, would be of some comfort.

Chaos is difficult to recall. That was my parents' house. When Tracy, Angie, and I arrived, I caned up the stairs and through the front door. The house had its familiar smell but resonated with tension and quiet. I remember the first hours were a pinball machine of hugging and clenching. I'd step ahead, and my sister would grab me, softly weeping, no words, and we'd stay that way, then I'd move to the kitchen and Ma would be there, grab my hand and hold it, rant under her breath, then we'd separate until the next pass. On and on through the house, back and forth, from person to person, all of us aimless and drifting until we'd find one another again in the hallway, by a window, or on the sundeck. A family breaking apart, reconfiguring, and breaking apart again, molecular, looking for its missing order. Mykol left us at one point and walked the gravel path through the nearby ravine, a tangle of trees, cutgrass, and dry creek bed where we'd played as kids. He found a broken beer bottle near the bridge, put it to his arm, and carved Rory's name.

My grandparents arrived at the house and joined the pacing. I was already downstairs most of the time and on the phone, calling all the numbers I could remember. Fill the house, I figured. Instead of twenty, make it five steps to find the next person you can lean on. With the rhythm established, the house stayed this way for weeks. Flowers everywhere. Food stacking in the freezer. The smell of coffee at all hours. Packages of cigarettes and Kleenex.

"I can't do it," Ma said to me the next morning. "The coroner is going to call with the toxicology results, but I can't do it."

"Don't worry," I said, "I'll take it."

Every time the phone rang, the house seized. I shuffled from wherever I happened to be and pawed for the receiver. Eventually the call came and filled me with numbers and chemistry I didn't totally understand, except for their consequence.

"Don't tell me," Ma said, "I don't want to hear about it right now."

It was difficult, but I kept the information to myself. I knew something about how relatively little was in Rory's system. I also knew which drug it was. The implications of what I knew weren't clear to me, not yet. The knowledge may have felt like carrying hot coals, but my parents weren't ready. Not until the funeral was over, perhaps. When she was up to it, which wouldn't take long, Ma would begin her ritual and get her hands on every scrap of information. Keeping it to myself gave her the right to choose her moment, and she deserved at least that much. It was a minor thing, but nothing seemed too minor.

The funeral was arranged, so we needed to make the calls. I sat on the floor in Rory's old bedroom with my sister. She opened my parents' thick, black address book to the letter A and read me the first name and phone number. I felt like a sniper. "Hi, it's Ryan Knighton calling. Yes, good to hear your voice, too. Yes, it's been a long time. I wish I was calling with better news, but. . . ." Again and again, "I've got some terrible news . . ." or "I hate to tell you this, but. . . ." Load, dial, fire, repeat. With each call, someone fell silent in my ear, at the other end of the line.

The intention here is not to cast myself as a hero. There's nothing heroic about helping. Plenty of difficulty was met head on by everybody, and it continues. I'm not alone. But I want the contrast to be clear. In recalling a life lived into blindness, I know now that Rory's death made me a different man and a different blind man. My eyes today are worse. Yet, somehow, today I'm far more at peace with seeing less. When Rory died, everything became easier; not perfect, but easier. I had been a young man in denial, one who resisted his diagnosis and its future at every turn. I'd mocked blindness, ignored it, camouflaged it, even accepted it, to a very minor degree. Rory's death, however, left a space, and that space demanded I become the kind of person I wanted to be: resolved, selfless, capable, any number of adjectives I'd let my blindness disfigure in me. Rory's absence made room to grow. If I'd been at war, it was more or less over. Whatever I'd been fighting didn't matter to me anymore. It was just too small.

Letting go of my sight, which is my past, has never been an intuitive process. What started in Pusan finished to a degree with Rory. More than anything, his death forced me to make room for a world that didn't revolve around my blindness. I miss things every day, but what are they? Objects. Phenomena with colour, depth, and shape. They have smells, tastes, textures, and weight. This world makes a lot of noise, and even more when I bump into its design. In the rain outside my window I hear the substance and size of what I can't see. Sure, I miss things, but Rory's death is the first time something in my world went missing. I thought I knew loss, but what did I know? Little. That's why, when we laid Rory to rest, I tried to put something to rest in me, too. Things grow smaller in the distance, and things disappear. Even blindness can. That's what I hope for. That's what I owe him and me.

The day before his funeral, several hours were set aside at the chapel for family to sit with Rory's body. Each by each, we came to say goodbye and to see him one last time. People say it's a good thing, to see a person one last time. It gives closure, they say. But what if you're blind? What does closure look like?

I didn't go to the viewing. The old me would have stayed home out of denial, as escape. But not anymore. Of my own choosing, I sat and smoked in the sun, on my back deck, and tried to remember what Rory looked like, how he moved, the plump feeling of his arm when I held it and he guided me. I listened to his voice. The person I said goodbye to that day was the one who, a week earlier, told me over the phone he was bored, just making pancakes, just wondering what I was up to. But the image I let go was from years before. It's difficult, but I can remember the sight of Rory's face when he was young. I don't really know what my brother looked like when he died and never will. Seeing him one last time wasn't necessary. In a way, I'd done that years ago. My other senses of him needed one last visit, though. No viewing could give me that, so I sat with Rory, on my deck, in my mind.

As for my parents and Mykol and Erin, they were going blind. I still feel for their extra loss. They had to let go of something they'd never see again, albeit just one sight, an immeasurable image we loved.

Seeing is itself touched with elegy. Reality seems to press its light into us, it is happening, but that's not the way things are. The eye can process only so many images per second, taking in sights the way a camera takes a series of stills. The reality we see is the sketchpad comics we made as kids, me and my brothers and sister. Draw a stickman taking a step on one page, and on the next draw that same figure, only his foot is slightly further ahead, and again on the next page, draw this figure, but with his foot on the ground. Flip through them quickly, and he appears to walk. That's the mechanics of the eye, too. We think we are seeing life as it happens, but pictures are missing. Moments disappear between the stills and make up our unwitnessed lives. To see is to miss things. Loss is always with us.

Seeing also takes time. Light travels at its pace, as do the signals from our retinas, passing from cells to nerves, and then, once within the brain, images are made. We move among them. But what we've seen has already happened out there, barely a moment ago, as a past we live within. The world we see is always gone.

I'm told that Rory's son, Gavin, looks more and more like his father every day. When Gavin is twenty-one, I won't know what that means. For now, I can piece together a picture of him from the memories of my little brother, from when we were kids. How strange to use memory to see what is in front of me today, to see what is missing.

In the summer of 2003, four years after Rory's death, Tracy

and I married. Many people must know this feeling. When you've been through what we have, the weight of what's behind can't help but push you forward and together, closer. Through it all, she stood beside my family and became part of its new order. I carry on as a stronger person because of her. Now and then my eyes throw a wrench in our plans, but nothing of a scale or significance worth really sweating about. People often ask me how we live together and what it's like to build blindness into an otherwise normal middle-class life. The truth is, it's hard to see. Blindness for us is mostly made of many small things. I reach for a glass but can't find it. I continue to talk to you over the table, looking for the glass with my hand. The moment I give up, Tracy nudges the glass to my fingers. It's so casual, the allowance she gives me to try and to fail, and it is so reflexive, her help when I need it. To learn how to live like this, together, took much time and patience. From where you sit, our way might not catch your eye. The exchange is so fluid and quick, like one of those moments in between the stills.

Without exaggeration or sentimentality, I can say Tracy is the greatest mystery of my disability. To live with me, she denies herself some pleasures, the kinds sight guarantees, and the kinds the sight of two people guarantees. This means, ultimately, she gives up some of who she is. How could I ask that of anyone? How could she agree? How does someone wake up each morning and choose to stay with blindness? I never did. How does she cope with a body even I want to leave? It's not my place or capacity to answer for her. But what I do know is this much.

A blind person and a sighted partner can come to an intimacy few are given. Imagine you only see the world through the eyes and the words of another. Many of our shared experiences are created by what Tracy chooses to narrate from the visual reality around us. Think about that. Relinquish your eyes, which means some of your consciousness, to the control of another person. Or claim that responsibility for yourself. I take in little other than what Tracy does. In this I am given to her, and she to me. It's both an alarming and rewarding way to live, tangled as a spliced being, a deeply bound physiology of one who looks out upon the world as two. That's startling when you first experience it and hard to let go. I've grown with another person as an extension of my own body and waking life. I don't mean this figuratively, either, no metaphor intended. Tracy is an extension of my body. To be as plain and true as I can, she sees for me, the way I would have wanted to.

Sacrifice has always been our problem and our solution. What Tracy gives up makes room for my blindness and, at the same time, enriches our bond. A poet I know once defined it this way: love, he said, is the compassionate understanding of the discord between the heart and the world. Tracy knows my discord, my blindness, pitch perfect. Her understanding comes from rare compassion, one without pity or martyrdom. My difficulty has always been to give back in kind. Some days I don't know how.

I'm told Tracy was something to see on our wedding day, but even I could have told you that. A butter-coloured gown and her hands full of chocolate-brown orchids. Her family gave me a dressy black cane for the occasion. As Tracy and I walked down the aisle, I swung it ahead for the two of us. Mykol stood by me as my best man, and Gavin carried the rings. After the ceremony, before dinner, my sister lit a candle for Rory and placed it on the table between Gavin and my parents. Once in a while its brightness cut through the blur of my eyes. Certainly I've known more than loss. So much more. All these people, they surround me, so strong and constant. Like light.

Jungle Fun

Two years ago I found myself on a small island, about a twenty-minute ferry ride from West Vancouver. Most of the island residents are hippies who sell nice soaps and project their egos into trees. Tracy had stayed in Vancouver with our dog and her own projects. I was on my own, except for the thirty-one other blind people I shacked up with.

I'd arrived at my first Gimp Camp. In the land of the blind, the one-eyed man is not king. He's a senior activities director. I know, I know. Don't call myself a gimp and don't call it a Gimp Camp. But I say it with pride. For three years I tried to sign up. The previous summer alone I'd failed to dial the camp's Vancouver office several times. I couldn't bring myself to enquire about available spaces. That's sort of why I wanted to go in the first place. True, we were going to swim and kayak and slam into one another a lot, the fun stuff, but, more importantly, I had a goal: I wanted to confront my fear, not of blindness, but of blind people.

First, I had some old camping issues to wrestle. I hadn't even unpacked my swim trunks before I was overcome with ghosts. Arriving at the lodge, I felt the same way I did at Cub Scout camp when I was a kid: I wanted to go home. Directly. Viscerally. I am not a camper, I realized, I am still a home-goer.

When I was seven or eight, at Campbell Valley's Cub Scout Jamboree, I wanted to go home because Lucas Ballard wet the bunk above me. The other five scouts I bunked with, strangers to each other's company, galvanized friendships around the accident. Not with me, though.

After the first night, from an academic perspective, it was all a matter of hardcore anthropology, really. The culture of Cabin #4 formed, like all cultures are formed, when the group rallied itself around a collective, symbolic killing, its common purpose and shared sense of camaraderie. Pick any historical example you like, from Gilgamesh to Christ to Communists. Make a scapegoat, and you make a people around it.

But Cabin #4 didn't hamstring Lucas for his moistened weakness—that would've been too cruel. Instead they tormented me all night about sleeping under Lucas's rusting mattress springs.

In the morning we marched to an obstacle course in the woods. Four pimply teenaged boys from the upper ranks of scoutdom had cooked up our course. I don't know how to explain it, but they seemed to have invested all their teen angst and sexual frustration in the design. It wasn't an obstacle course per se; it was retribution, pure, private, poisonous retribution for whatever it is that junior high school does to pimply-faced boys who earn badges for good mapmaking skills. When we arrived, one of the older scouts told us to wait in line for a few more minutes.

"We're not done hosing yet," he explained, and ran back into the woods, dragging a thick green garden hose after him. I could hear other boys, out of sight, too, cackling and hooting with cracked, pubescent voices. The only other sound was water, lots of water spraying.

What needs hosing down in an obstacle course? Some of us speculated. Others kept a dignified silence and tried to keep nervous stomachs from barfing up handfuls of eggs and porridge. Myself, I imagined the older scouts rinsing all the blood off the obstacles, the blood from the previous week's campers. In my mind I saw carnage and twisted, painful faces, boys who'd impaled themselves on tree branches as they scrambled over logs, others grinding their knees to the bone as they crawled under a stretch of low brush tangled with razor wire. And then the free-for-all, like a war movie. I imagined dozens of cub scouts trampling to the finish line, the unfortunate and weak dropping to their knees or tripping on their poorly tied shoelaces, stomped by a herd of do-gooders who know ten practical uses for human hair. Blood. It was definitely blood they had hoses to deal with.

Mine was only an approximation of what we found. While it's true I did eventually see boys clambering over logs, dropping out of trees, breaking a leg or two, and I did see a violent stampede for the finish, the hoses weren't for the blood. They were for the mud. The entire obstacle course was set within an expansive muck that came up to our knees. We crawled in it, fell in it, swallowed it, flung it and, supposedly, enjoyed it. The name they'd given this inspiriting camp activity was "jungle fun."

Our reward for crossing the finish line was a long, icy blast from Gary and Todd, the worst of the older scouts who assisted the phantom adult camp directors. The finish line looked like a Vietnam demonstration, dozens of boys lined up, hands over their faces, hosed by our two budding riot police.

Cabin #4 was quiet that night. Even though we didn't understand anthropology or know how to say it, we knew in our hearts we were all to be sacrificed here. We wanted to go home early. We'd only experienced the first twenty-four hours of our summer. Lucas cried a lot.

I can't say my arrival at blind camp was nearly as dramatic or wet. Nevertheless, once again I wanted to go home before the fun started. Maybe even earlier. The thought had crossed my mind before I'd signed up, too.

In order to secure my place among the other blind campers, I'd had to register at the Vancouver office of the Canadian National Institute for the Blind. They'd long ago moved shop from the old, military-style barracks into a sterile, hospital-like building. I don't know what they do for blind folks all day long, and I've never mustered much enthusiasm for trekking down to find out. A lot of blind people are usually there, and that's enough to keep me away. I'm certain many of them are super folks, but I can still see just enough to make out some of the faces there, and the shuffling bodies, and the confusion in the hallways. I can't run, but if I could, I couldn't run from that fast enough. I hoped confinement to an island with my people might show me something about them and why I react this way.

Marla, the lodge's director, helped me register for camp once I'd found the courage to call and to make my way to the new CNIB digs. She was short and sighted, square and frazzled. Her shoulder-length gray hair frayed in every direction. She also wore those white, clunky shoes, the ones only nurses know where to buy. We walked to her office and sat together at her desk long enough for me to piece together that much of her appearance.

What she saw, primarily, was a jittery blind man who sweated a great deal. That's what always happened to me at the CNIB. I could do nothing but sweat an anxious, clammy sweat. Good campfire retardant.

"The only thing we have to do," she said, "is fill out this medical form. Then you can pay the fee, and you're set for camp. Good stuff?"

On her desk she dropped the weight of a thick application booklet.

"Tremendous," I agreed.

"The medical form is a bit long. Should I read it to you and help you fill it out? Or, if you like, you can take it home and have someone help you, then bring it back tomorrow."

I felt a fresh surge of sweat at the thought of a return trip to the CNIB. At this rate, I wouldn't make it to camp without dying of dehydration. "Let's do it now, " I said.

Marla filled out my particulars, my name and address, then got to the meat of the book we called a form.

"Now," she began, turning to page two, "there's a list of medical details we need to establish. They're just yes or no answers. Good stuff?"

"Terrific."

"Okay, do you have some sight?"

"Yes."

"Night vision?"

"No."

"Tunnel vision?"

"Barely. In one eye. About one percent works."

"Do you use a cane, a dog?"

"Yes and no."

"Do you need a personal guide?"

"No. But I like them. Especially when driving."

"I think," Marla paused, "I can check a bunch of these off quickly. Let's see, you aren't in a wheelchair, you are not deaf, you don't have behavioural problems. Right?"

Problems? I wasn't sure if sweating or a paralysing fear of blind people would count, so I let the question pass. "No, don't think so."

"You don't need twenty-four-hour care, no night attendant, no assistance with personal hygiene, bathroom equipment, no wheelchair . . ."

Her list continued, as did my concern. I knew I would be partnered with somebody in a room at the lodge. Unfortunately, I began to wonder what that person would be like. The picture Marla suggested wasn't comforting. According to her list, I could be sleeping next to a shell of a body with no arms or legs, strapped inside an oxygen tent, with an on-call surgical team hanging out in the corner of our room, just in case. They would accompany us on our canoe trips, too, administering shots and applying ointments when necessary.

"Do you have asthma?" Marla asked.

"Nope."

"Any STD's, insomnia, food allergies, or heart trouble?"

The portrait of my bunkmate refined itself. Not only would he complain about the noise made by his private surgical team, he'd complain about the clap, arrhythmia, and lactose intolerance keeping him up at night.

"No to them all."

"Nightmares?" she added.

"Plenty."

"Have you ever been hospitalized for depression, violence, suicide, or psychotic episodes?"

I shook my head no, hoping sweat wouldn't fly from my face.

"What about medications? Do you take any medications?"

"Can I bring a stash?"

"Good stuff," she giggled, and then leaned across her desk, as if about to confide in me something about her own phar-maceutical preferences.

"Sorry," she whispered, "I have to ask this, but do you, I mean, are you a bed wetter?"

I was seven years old again. Lucas Ballard would be my blind camp bunkmate, the poor guy. What the hell could have happened to leave him in such a maimed state? Maybe the obstacle course really did him in.

"No," I admitted, "not in a while."

Marla finished the form with me, and a half an hour later I signed myself up for camp.

"One other thing, " she added. "Do you wish to make this information available to other campers?"

"Huh?"

"In the past, some have asked if they can find out more

information about their roommates before choosing them. If people agree to make the information available, we see no problem with that."

I remembered from my high school sports experiences how captains picked their teammates one at a time, a system that left a few poor kids last to be chosen, and thereby consolidated public opinion that, yes, indeed, Derek, Sandy, and Eugene were exceedingly lame. Would that happen here too, on an island retreat for the disabled? We'd be down to the final three and some über-jock blind man would be picking his bunkmate.

"I read Ryan's just sweaty, so I think he's okay. Bill and Mindy are both asthmatics. That's not so bad, I guess. Marla, could you read Bill's record again? I think he checked off bed wetter, but I can't remember."

Darwinism even applies within a group of blind people. But I let it go. I didn't want to cause trouble so soon.

"Sure," I agreed, "why not let it all hang out?"

"Good stuff."

Tracy took me out for breakfast the day I left for camp. She would drop me off at the CNIB afterward, where I would catch the bus Marla had arranged to transport a number of campers to the island. At the restaurant I poked at my eggs and sausage with the solemnity of a man about to begin his prison sentence. What would I have in common with anybody other than an inability to see well? The deaf, unlike the blind, have their own culture. They have a shared language. Culture and identity begin there. But what do the blind share

other than an indifference towards sunsets? Anything?
Worse, would the camp force us to make arts and crafts?
Would there be jungle fun? Tracy, always thoughtful, had
tucked a fresh bottle of Irish whiskey into my suitcase.

"If you have to sing around the campfire," she reasoned,
"you'd best be lubricated."

When she dropped me off at the CNIB, Jason, one of the
four camp counselors, met me at the door. Normally, he said,
there would be at least eight counselors, but funding cuts
were such that the lodge could only afford four counselors for
all thirty-one campers. This should be fun, I thought, perking
up a little. Low supervision for the low of vision.

Jason, like the other employees, was in his early twenties,
friendly, helpful, and, unlike the others, Green Giant–large.
His hand swallowed mine when we shook them. When he
said it was nice to meet me, his voice came from a mouth
somewhere above my eyebrows.

He guided me to a chair in a lounge area where two other
campers waited. He left us and resumed his post at the door.
Jason hadn't said a word, and my nod of thanks for the guidance maintained the silence. Either both campers had agreed
through ESP to pretend I wasn't there, or neither had any
idea I was waiting with them. Great, I thought. Maybe I could
pull this off all week. Don't make a sound, and nobody will
know I'm here.

Later I would learn that the two people sitting across from
me were Eddie and Cheryl. Eddie was in his mid-twenties.
His only distinguishing feature, from what I could tell, was a

large pair of 1970s-style headphones clamped to his head. Amphetamine-crazed metal pleased him. During our week at camp, he never seemed to take the headphones off.

Near him sat Cheryl, a private and pleasant young woman. She suffered some sort of occasional Tourette's or linguistic tick, as well as blindness. Every once in a while she'd erupt, shouting one of two words—"f-f-f-f-f-f-fuggin" or "sh-sh-sh-shimbles." I don't know what they meant. I doubt if she did, either. Otherwise, she was soft-spoken and, from what I could guess, maybe had a closed, worried expression. Sitting across from me, she looked tight-lipped and pensive. Or something.

It may have been the case that both Eddie and Cheryl knew nothing of the other's presence, too. We waited, all three of us mute, while I sweated something awful.

Then Martin arrived. Or maybe I should say Martin's relentless jabber arrived. Jason guided Martin to the lounge, but I heard his voice well in advance.

"This is gonna be some camp, Jason. You're new this year, right? It's some fun, and the ladies, oh, the ladies are always the highlight, my friend. You single? Catch as catch can, as they say. I brought a radio this year in case I'll be entertaining in my room. Nudge, nudge, wink, wink, as they say, eh? You like the Python? Lots of oldies, that's what I like. Not the ladies. I mean tunes. They just don't write them like they used to. I collect songs about driving truck. 'Truckin,' now that's a song."

Martin was my age and was desperate to get laid at blind camp. A tradition existed of past campers coming here, hook-ing up and sometimes marrying. Imagine a hybrid of *Gilligan's Island* and *The Love Boat,* but everybody has a stick.

Jason guided Martin into the lounge and sat him on a chair next to Cheryl. Eddie remained on the other side of her, and I sat across the room from them all, cloaked in quiet. When Eddie heard Martin's soliloquy coming down the hall, he began to beam.

"Martin? Martin-o, the Martinmeister? Is that you, man? The Don Martin? Marty the Martini Maker?"

"Who's that?" Martin asked, taking his seat.

"It's me, Eddie! Eddie from Kamloops!"

"Heavy Eddie Metal!" Martin cheered. "How the hell are you!"

"I'm great, man. Brought my tunes with me."

"Me, too," said Martin. "You never know when you'll need some mood music."

"Divine Blade!" Eddie shrieked. "Hey! Hey! Have you heard Divine Blade? They rock and roll, man. Totally rawk!"

"I wonder who else is coming this year?" Martin said.

"Sh-sh-sh-shimbles."

"Cheryl!"

Old friends began to catch up. I doubt, though, Cheryl was so thrilled. Like me, she'd done her best to keep out of sight from Eddie and Martin. I mean, keep quiet, or whatever the phrase would be.

Most of the campers were making their way to the island under their own steam, so Jason drove a van, just six of us and our luggage stuffed inside. Perhaps spying my sweaty condition, Jason offered me the front seat near the air vents. Or maybe he sensed that, like him, I was new to this scene.

In the back sat Cheryl, Eddie, and Martin, joined by Liza and Dick, a couple who'd met at the camp twenty years earlier and married. They returned every year.

Dick had a little residual sight, maybe as much as I did, but he also had some nerve damage that accentuated his shuffling step and made him stutter. Once he'd been a helicopter pilot who crashed while fighting forest fires, his crash caused by his own misjudgement, and his misjudgement caused by eight days straight of flying sixteen-hour shifts.

Despite all Dick's years of flying and his years before that of driving a long-haul truck, a fact that tickled Martin to no end, Dick was calm and deliberate, even happily slow in manner. It interested me that he betrayed no frustration. He was a man who once spent the majority of his time moving at high speeds, then was forced to live at the opposite pace. Surprisingly, he seemed without urgency or anger. His partner, Liza, was kind and genuine and perky. Mostly strange, though.

"Ryan," she said at one point during the drive and grabbed for my shoulder from the back seat. When she found me, she beat my shoulder like an elevator call button. "Ryan," tap, tap, tap. "Ryan," tap, tap.

"Yes, Liza?"

"You know what, you should play along with me and Dick this week. We have this game we used to play at camp. Ever since we were married, we play it at home, too."

"What's the game?" I asked. I tried not to imagine anything they played at home.

"Well," she began, and tweaked her voice up a pitch, like a little girl. "Dick and I have this thing. We have cats, lots of cats. Both of us love cats. Sometimes we take Blinky when we walk to the mall for a coffee and a sausage roll. Anyway, we have this game, and what happens is people will be talking, and someone might say something like, 'Who spilled the salt?' Somebody will go to answer, and they'll say, 'Oh, I think it was—' That's when Dick and I sing together, 'Yyooooour caaaaat.'"

They did it, in harmony.

"It's fun," she explained. "Want to play this week?"

I felt I had to say yes, only because I didn't understand. Liza made me practise harmonizing a couple of times before we arrived at camp. I still don't know what the game meant or why they did it. Why we did it.

When we arrived at the lodge, I discovered a benevolent fact. Thirty-one campers meant one person had to bunk alone. Jason asked if I'd mind, since everybody else had already paired off with old friends. I tried not to nod too enthusiastically. Sleeping alone guaranteed that nobody could wet the bunk above me.

At breakfast the next morning, Jason announced we'd have a fire drill in an hour, or maybe in two hours. He had a good feel for the timing of blind people. We have one speed, and it's somewhere between dawdle and mosey.

"The fire drill is an insurance thing," he explained, "but no big deal, really. It's timed, too, so it shouldn't take long."

Although more like a Spartan dormitory than anything else, the lodge had a spacious wooden dining hall with generous windows that looked out over our dirty bay. The dock was out there somewhere, several canoes and paddleboats tied to it. I bet we made the locals plenty nervous when we took to the water near their yachts.

For meals and happy hour we sat at six large, round tables, five or six campers at each. We were served by two chipper young students who, like me, wanted to go home. I couldn't blame them. Somehow they managed to feign cheer even when helping the table of shameless, nit-picking yobs, the ones I thought of as the Aristocrats. These people mistook our camp for a private resort and mistook themselves for a blind elite who deserved to look down upon the rest of us. I can still hear them.

"Oh, Miss! Where are the servers? I've been waiting for ten minutes? Miss! Miss! Can you remove the onions from my salad? I said no onions. Can you cool my soup with an ice cube? Can you pick the seeds off my bread? When you're done, can you take those seeds, plant them, grow wheat, mill it, and bake some seedless loaves before serving me another onion sandwich?"

Of Eddie and Cheryl and others, me included, the Aristocrats often commiserated how young blind people today have it too easy. We stay home, live with our parents, collect government money, and refuse to integrate ourselves into the sighted world. Such helplessness, the Aristocrats complained, when so many technologies and opportunities are practically given away. "In our day, we had to fend for ourselves and learn how to . . ."

The Aristocrats didn't like it, but not everything was done

for the campers. For one thing, we fetched our own coffee from the large steel urns the students kept topped up throughout the day. The sugar and cream station was a massacre of dirty spoons, half-emptied sweetener packets, puddles of honey and half-and-half, and a variety of solids I felt but couldn't identify. Everything fused to everything else. If the world ended today, centuries from now some future people might discover that coffee station and take it for a significant midden of a very unkempt people. But we managed. We plunged our hands into the primordial muck and hoped to find what we needed.

We also ate waffles every morning, except on the days we had pancakes. A large syrup jug rested in the middle of each table. Campers were on their own to pour and hope for the best. From all indications, my chair had been sticky since 1983.

On fire drill day, my comrades at the breakfast table included Liza and Dick. "Let me know when I've got enough syrup," Liza asked her hubby and began to pour. As she did, they both stared out the windows, or what would be out the windows if they could have seen through them. When Dick thought Liza had poured enough, he said so, and she stopped, sort of. Neither seemed to care if he was right. They'd gone through the ritual of good table manners and that was enough to satisfy. The result, which spilled over the plate and pooled a bit around my juice glass, was irrelevant.

The syrup business was a good lesson for me. I actually joined in the fun for once. We all did it. We'd ask each other for help, pretend to give it, then carry on, thanking our helpful fellow camper as we wiped our sticky hands on the sticky tablecloth. It was a gentle anarchy, a dysfunctional politeness, and it was ours. Sweet.

These details suggest something about how Jason's fire drill would proceed. Modern dance troupes could only be in awe of its choreography. The drill could only be about as weird as modern dance, too.

Martin and another camper, Kevin, were chummy from previous years. They were both notably alarmed when Jason announced the oncoming safety exercise, particularly Kevin, who had a frantic manner most of the time and a needy, high-pitched voice to match. I could hear them at the table next to mine, where Jason also ate his breakfast. Kevin prodded Jason relentlessly.

"You're gonna let us know when the fire drill is, right? You're gonna let us know, right?"

Part of Kevin's frenetic way was to use up extra energy repeating himself.

"For sure," Jason said, for the fifth or sixth time, "not to worry. You'll know when it's coming."

"Heh, heh, heh," Martin feigned a chuckle. "Yep, heh, heh, we wouldn't want the alarm to just go off. It might frighten people. Heh, heh. Wouldn't want that."

"Don't worry," Jason said. "I wouldn't think of it. Everything will be clear when we get around to—"

Kevin asserted himself. "Alarms. I don't like alarms. That's all I'm saying. I don't like alarms." He sounded as if he'd just discovered this about himself, and the fact surprised him.

"Me neither!" Martin added, equally surprised.

"Wouldn't know what to do," Kevin said. "Wouldn't know how to do it, either."

Martin grunted in agreement. "It could be real. How would we know?"

"That's the worst," Kevin agreed. "Real alarms are the worst."

The alarmists continued while the others at their table picked up a new topic of conversation, although not a fresh one. Breakfast chit-chat focused on one of several things. Lots of campers liked to compare medications and personal data about which ones worked better than others for what symptoms, everything from ulcers to depression to thyroid malfunction. Then there was the gossip. Which campers liked which campers, which CNIB case workers were better than others, which regions had the best programs for kitchen skills, afternoon bingo, or white-water rafting. But people mostly talked meds. During breakfast the four counselors distributed a variety of drugs. The stuff was all prescription and necessary, and more pills than I've ever encountered outside a pharmacy or a good rave. I'm talking about a plastic baggy of gel capsules, and that was sometimes for just one person's morning intake. They were like bean bags, these handouts.

That, I think, pulled some facts into focus. Take Liza and Dick, for instance. Punctuating other people's sentences with a harmony of "your cat" probably is a truckload of fun with that much chemistry in your system.

But I also discerned something better than before, a fact I'd neglected. In the cleanliness of my own blood, I felt some of my fortune and privilege. I may be blind, but I don't cope with brain damage, weak organs, psychological trauma, or a myriad of other unimaginables along with it. Mine is a kind of aristocracy, too, if I'm not careful. I'm merely blind, the stock model, and, in addition, I have a wisp of low-functioning sight. That would have been enough to radically change several lives around my table.

"Are we doing the drill now?" Kevin asked.

"It's been five minutes," Jason said. "Everybody's still eating."

"I just thought it might be coming. I want to be ready. You know, for the alarm."

Jason and the other three counselors had misplaced the alarm keys, after all. They wouldn't be able to shut it off if they turned it on, so a new plan was struck. I think Kevin gasped. It was decided we'd all go back to our rooms and wait until we heard Jason's cue. He'd shout from his post downstairs, "Fire! Fire!" and then the drill would be on.

"Can you not shout it too, you know, loud?" Martin asked.

Kevin demonstrated. "Maybe just, 'Fire! Fire!' That would be enough, don't you think?"

After breakfast, everybody caned back to their rooms and shut their doors. On the way, much conversation filled the halls about who would lead whom, how roommates would find one another when we reached the safety of the lawn, and so on. Once in our rooms, the building silent, the tension grew. This wasn't just an insurance exercise. This was on par with semifinals at the World Cup Fire Drill.

Then the call came. We heard Jason's homemade alarm from downstairs, and we were off.

Doors shot open and slammed shut, canes dropped to the floor, keys scraped, and locks locked. For some reason, we'd tacitly agreed that doors were to be secured. Jason shouted from one end of the hall, downstairs.

"No, no, don't worry about the locks! Just go!"

"I'm not leaving my walkman if I can't lock the door," Eddie shouted back. I heard him open his door and go back inside to fetch Divine Blade.

"I forgot my coat," Cheryl said. "F-f-f-f-fuggen." Back into her room she went.

"Oh, good idea, Cheryl," Liza chirped, "it's raining." Back she went to her room with Dick leading the way.

"Just go!" Jason shouted. "This is a fire drill, folks! We won't be outside long!"

"I'll wait for Eddie," Martin said, hanging around his door.

Kevin was already well down the hall, but he decided he'd wait for Eddie, too. He caned his way back while Martin guided, saying, "I'm over here, you're warm, you're getting warmer." Had it been a real fire, Kevin's warmth would have been severe.

"Hey, Jason," Kevin called. "I meant to ask if you think Martin and I could switch roommates?"

"Forget it," Jason said. "Fire drill's over. It took too long. We have to do it again. This time everybody have your coats on and be ready to go when I shout fire. Back into your rooms, please, and let's try it again."

Back into the gates we went and prepared for a second race. When Jason made his alarm noise, we threw open our doors, shot from our rooms, and again played with the locks.

"No locks," Jason hollered, "abandon all locking and go!"

We actually made it down the hall towards the stairs, a mass of canes and zigzagging campers, all of us swinging, stopping, going, knocking into one another and then the stairs, a slow funnel like a blocked artery. Most campers descended on either side of the staircase, following the handrails, making a trickling line of campers in single file. A few people like me, the ones with a little sight, barreled down the middle of the mostly empty stairwell. In the chaos, nobody listened to Jason.

"You're going the wrong way," he shouted.

He and the other counselors had forgotten one key fire drill element. None of us knew where the closest exit was. We were heading, all of us, to the dining hall and the only exit we knew.

"Go to the other end, go back the other way," he pleaded.

I called back to the crowd on the stairs. "I think Jason wants us to turn around, guys."

Everybody stopped.

"And go where?" Dick asked.

"I dunno," I said. "Where are we going?"

"The emergency exit is at the other end of the hall!" Jason said.

My sense of timing isn't the most precise, but I think, in a real fire, we'd have all baked to death by then.

"Where at the end?" Martin asked. "I don't know what you mean when you say at the end."

Jason probably gestured. "You know, that way, the end of the hall. Just there."

"Sh-sh-sh-shimbles."

"Yeah, but where at the end?" Kevin asked.

Dick clarified. "Is the emergency door on the left or right?"

I guessed it was on the left, but a couple of campers disagreed.

"No," Jason said, "that's Eddie's room."

"I locked my door," Eddie said. "We can't go that way."

I thought Jason was going to melt on the spot. "Here," he conceded, "how about I just show you guys where it is and if there's a fire, promise to use that door, okay?"

That seemed reasonable to everybody. We followed him down the hall and discovered a new door. Everybody got the hang of how to open it and run for our lives.

All of this points to one thing I admire about blindness and the blind. We have an incomparable ability to throw a wrench in bureaucracy, whether we mean to or not. Our bodies are collectively so idiosyncratic and uncooperative, as are some of our personalities, that we don't lend ourselves well to goals like efficiency and standardization. I mean, you can't standardize the movements of this many blind people, and you can't take anything about us for granted, either. That's the bureaucratic goal, right? We went through the insurance drill so that the insurers could assume all the blind folks knew how to get out of the building. As if. I doubt if any of us could have left the building the same way twice. It was a gentle, even an unintentional, anarchy.

Not all mornings began with such a scene. In fact, Tai Chi was the main morning activity during camp. I took a liking to

Tai Chi. Jesus, no, I didn't do it, but I enjoyed my coffee at
the far end of the dining hall while a handful of others, down
at the opposite end, did their best to strike a pose. From
where I sat, I could squeeze bits of the action into view.
Carson, our novice, led the show. He was a fellow camper and
one of my favourite people.

"Now, make a wing," Carson said one morning, "but make
it high-up and flat, like a tipping sailboat."

Carson likely saw at some point in his life. The imagery he
used suggested as much. I noticed he took a lot of analogies
from the ocean. I wondered if he'd lost his sight in a boating
accident or something. Our Poseidon. I imagined birds nib-
bling at his eyes. Hitchcocky stuff.

To describe a Tai Chi move to newcomers, blind newcomers, is difficult. Inkblots would be a similar challenge to put
into words. Carson hadn't thought his lessons through. Not
everybody had seen a sailboat, let alone the tipping kind.
Carson had to bust out the technical manual and try again.

"Or think of it this way," he said. "Take your right hand,
bend at the elbow and turn it inward at the wrist and open
your fingers, like a starfish, and then, holding your elbow up
as high as you can, pull a hand towards you, the right one,
like you are calling somebody, but keep the hand and arm
parallel to your chest, more like you are raking than calling
somebody, maybe. Now turn your wrist and swim, extending
the arm out, follow through, always follow through, and
return and swim out again and . . ."

A half a dozen people contorted. They looked like they'd
fallen out of trees and busted their elbows and shoulders.

Carson had said swim, but few did. Some updated the chicken dance, others went fly fishing, and Eddie broke into an impromptu round of shadow boxing. Carson hadn't said anything about how fast the arm should go, so Eddie's pace went rapid-fire, a rhythm to match his morning dose of Van Halen. Liza's arm slowly stirred a pot of soup.

While all this was happening, Carson's lower body maintained an elegant pose, angled but relaxed. His students, however, ignored everything but their flapping. Some remained rigid, while others slouched into their normal bad postures. Eddie bent low at the knees, it appeared, with his legs wide apart, going for a lead singer crotch-shot, the kind struck before belting a high note.

I guess if you don't mention it to the blind, it isn't there. If you give the upper part of me guidance, the rest of me wouldn't know what to do. You'd think Carson, and the rest of us, would be conscious of such things with one another. Nope.

I expected, of all places in the world, this would be the one where sighted habits were dropped. They weren't. People sat around the breakfast tables and spoke to one another without identifying themselves or whom they meant to address. Cheryl might have asked something like, "Are you going to glue macaroni owls at the crafts table this afternoon?" Everybody would carry on chewing until somebody said the obligatory, "Are you talking to me?" All six dining tables sounded like a rehearsal from *Taxi Driver*. You talking to me? You talking to me?

It happened in the halls, too. Cruising around the lodge, its disorienting design, if we heard someone approaching, we said hello, but never, "Hello, it's Martin," or "Hello, it's Eddie." Even I forgot to add my name to my voice. The hallways echoed with a casual anthem: "Who's there?" All day and night, "Who's that?" and "Who's there?" If you hear the questions often enough, you begin to wonder at the depth of the answer. I don't know, I wanted to say. I don't know who's here. Who are we? Who are you? Could any of us really say?

Likewise, you'd think of all places in the world, this one would have been gesture-free. Nope. Everybody, me included, carried on flagging and pointing, and as you'd expect, none of us followed. We were so used to living with sighted people that we couldn't even be blind with one another.

Carson, from what I could tell, was the only one who avoided any of the above. Sometimes he avoided answering anything. Beyond his morning Tai Chi class, the guy was basically a ghost, walking the beach alone, or hanging out quietly on the edge of a chatty group, just listening. His self-reliance was a likeable trait. Enviable, even. Something in his character, some core resignation to his blindness, carried him. He maintained an eerie peace I wish I could know, a peace without irony, cynicism, or victimization propping it up. Those were the defences of choice for most people I met. Me, too.

While it's fair to say Carson kept to himself, unlike me, he didn't hide from the group in his room. His tactics differed and weren't born of fear. Within days I was running out of strategies to avoid people. Soon I borrowed one from Eddie. Headphones. I wore my walkman when I wanted to be left alone. It could have been surgically attached to my ears, I wore it so much during the first few days.

Initially I kept the sound off. I thought I'd developed a great way to say to people that I wasn't available. What I failed to see was the obvious. Nobody saw the headset, so conversations continued to follow me around the lodge and down to the beach.

To avoid everybody in a fresh fashion, I walked down to the lodge's dock for a swim one afternoon. It was raining, so I figured I'd be on my own for as long as I could stand the frigid water and whatever creepy stuff brushed against my toes. When I reached the end of the dock's wooden planks, I heard an extra set of footsteps behind me. They were Carson's. I asked if he came for a swim, but he said he didn't know how. He thought he'd just listen. And he did. Not a word passed between us. He likes to listen, that's all. I hoped one day to learn how to do that, too.

Seamus was my other pal. I first met Seamus, and took a liking to him, on our third day. A bunch of us joined Jason that afternoon for an annual camp highlight. We drove across the island to touch the big tree. It really was a big tree. Eight of us circled it. Then we all touched it. Good trip. Felt good, like a big tree, in fact.

Avoiding Seamus would have been hard. He loved to talk. More than that, he loved to tell you what was happening right here and now in the realm of the brutally obvious. On our way to the tree he sat in the back of the van and lobbed all his observations and descriptions at me.

"Hey, Ryan," he said, "how's the front seat?"

That wasn't small talk for Seamus. He overwhelmed it with curiosity, like he'd just discovered I'd once been clinically dead and now he needed to know how the experience measured up.

"The front seat is good, Seamus."

According to the counselors, Seamus was a camp regular and diehard. He squirreled away a little money every month, not an easy feat with a disability pension, to make the annual trip to camp. Seamus was perhaps in his fifties, but due to other conditions related to his blindness, his mental development had arrested around the age of six, maybe. From what I could determine, he had salt-and-pepper hair and was easily rattled. The only cure for his anxiety was the same as anybody's. He talked.

"Yep," he continued, "it's one good seat. I sat there last year. A really good front seat. Nice. This seat isn't so bad. I like it. I get to sit with two people, but you only sit with one. You got the window open?"

"Uh, nope."

"The window is good. I like wind. Wind, window. Wind and window—hey, they're almost the same. It's a good seat, Ryan. I sat there last year, you know."

"I'm sorry, Seamus. Did I take your spot?"

I'd had an autistic student freak once when I borrowed his pen. Seamus's condition wasn't clear to me, so I worried I'd upset some natural order. My concern baffled him.

"No, it's not my seat," he said, as if I'd picked it up and handed it to him. "It's your seat. This, this is my seat, in the back. You're sitting in the front seat, Ryan. That's your seat."

I didn't know what else to do or how to carry a conversation with him. Didn't matter, though. Seamus carried it for us, taking an inventory of all the possible subjects from the immediate environment. Troubled by a lull in dialogue, he narrated what was happening around him, so that you could pick something from his collection to talk about, be it an ashtray, temperature, funny sounds, what your name rhymed with, whatever he could find. He was an unrivaled surveyor of reality's lesser phenomena.

"Well," he continued, sensing our pause, "yep, the front seat, a good one. Ryan's in the front, and Jason's driving. We're driving together, and I'm in the back. Hey, the air conditioning is on, right, Jason?"

"Yep, it's on."

"It's good air conditioning, eh?"

"Works well."

"Are you cold, Ryan?"

"Nope, just cool."

"Air conditioning, air is con-di-tioning, ing-a-ling. It's a song! It's keeping us cool on our way to the big tree. Me, too, way back here. I'm sitting back here, Ryan. Yep, here we are, cool in the van and driving to the big tree. I've got my sandals on. Ryan's in the front seat, and Jason's in the—hey, I sat there last year, Ryan, but now you're sitting there. It's a nice seat, eh?"

And so on, until we arrived at the big tree and touched it.

Seamus irritated most campers, but something happened to me after fifteen minutes of listening to his consciousness. His effect switched from annoying to, I don't know, something like spiritual. His inventory of every moment caused a mild trance-like state in me. Comfort comes of describing what's happening all the time. I guess, in a way, it felt like the old days when I could relax my focus and idly look around. Seamus did it for all of us. Seamus looked around with words.

Some of the Aristocrats had no patience for him. They thought much of his constant difficulty and banter was a show for attention, not a medical reality. The Aristocrats were our right-wing equivalent of people who worry that somebody isn't really disabled, or disabled enough, only abusing the system for its perks. It happens. I've been accused by sighted people of not being blind enough for whatever it is blindness gets me. Like what, I don't know.

But to have carried on Seamus's epic monologues and to have needed the amount of help he did was an immense labour. If it was deliberate and unnecessary, wow. Christ, if I'd tried to pull it off, the perks would have to be pretty blue chip to have justified the effort. Having a counselor help me unlock my room doesn't strike me as cashing in on the lottery of personal aid, nor as an incentive to have recited "left foot, right foot, left foot," while we walked to the big tree. I'll never understand those who accuse disabled folks of milking their status.

What I liked even more about Seamus, more than his narration, was his lack of self-consciousness. No matter how much help or what kind of help he needed, no matter how many groans came from the Aristocrats, he asked for assistance, was unapologetic, and displayed no shame. We were the ones who were embarrassed for him, some of us, sometimes, but not him. That bugged the hell out of the Aristocrats.

I think they didn't want the association of Seamus as a peer in blindness. He made them look bad or feel awkward about themselves. He defined how they might or could one day appear to the sighted. Maybe a little of that identification, that fear, had once been in me, too. Maybe that had been part of my anxiety about other blind people to begin with. I didn't want them defining me.

Seamus's room was across the hall from mine. If his roommate wasn't with him—poetic justice dictated that to be Martin—Seamus was easily disoriented by the lodge's maze-like design. Half the time he tried his key in my door. Because I was often in my room, keeping dry and calm, I redirected him. Otherwise he would have spent, and did, a frightening amount of time trying and retrying his key in my lock.

"Seamus, your room is across the hall."

"Martin? Is that you? I can't get my key to work."

"No, Seamus, it's Ryan."

"Hey, Ryan! How's it going? Did you make a candle today? What are you doing in my room?"

"This is my room, Seamus. Yours is across the hall."

"I can't get my key to work. Maybe I have the wrong one. Do you have my key?"

"Your key doesn't work because this is my room."

"Oh. I see. This is your room." Seamus began to drown in confusion. Something in the world defied the laws of physics. "I don't mind if you're in my room now, but where's my stuff? Did Jason move my stuff?"

Sometimes the easiest way to help Seamus was the wrong one.

"Yeah, Seamus, Jason moved your stuff across the hall. Martin's, too."

"But I don't have a key for that room."

"Jason said your old key will work fine. Give it a try."

I heard him cross the hall and the deadbolt unlock. Martin had left his radio on, the volume loud. He'd tuned it to an oldies station, for the ladies at camp who were into that kind of groove. Johnny Cash filled the hallway as Seamus opened the door.

"It worked, Ryan! Okay, gonna go into my new room now. Now I've got to make sure all my stuff is here. I'm gonna go into the room now and shut the door and check all my stuff. Okay!?"

I called back, through the door, "You betcha, Seamus."

"Here I go. Gotta lock the door behind me. Here I go . . ."

One morning Seamus appeared well before sunrise. I woke to his key scratching in my lock and started up our routine.

"No, Seamus. It's my room, Ryan's room, yours is across the hall."

"Who's-ssat?"

Seamus sounded upset. Different.

"Ryan. It's Ryan, Seamus. Your room is—"

"Ryan? I canned find my deef! I canned find dem."

"Your teeth?"

"My deef."

"You want some help?"

"Yesh, pleash."

I got out of bed and opened the door. There stood Seamus in his pajamas with his cane. No teeth. I couldn't see that they were missing, but I could hear it.

We walked to the common bathroom, the last place he could recall wearing them, and began the search. Because it was so early, I decided not to get Jason up. Maybe the dentures were somewhere obvious. Two blind guys began their search for a pair of teeth. We felt for them. Everywhere.

Now that he had some help, the teeth didn't seem to matter to Seamus so much, and his panic dissipated. I touched shelves and countertops while Seamus wiped the bathroom floor with his hands. He chatted affably all the while.

"Do you have an elecdric rayshor?" he asked.

"Nope. Just a regular one."

"I'm nod allowed do have one. Do you like id bedder?"

"Yep."

"I'm nod allowed do have one, bud I've god a nyshe elecdric rayshor. And afder shave called Brud. I like Brud. Wanna shmell?"

"Maybe after we find your teeth."

"Okay. Hey, maybe I can dry your rayshor and you can dry mine. Do you like elecdric rayshors?"

We carried on until we'd fingered every surface of the washroom. Seamus's worry was pretty much gone, too, as if he couldn't care less if he ever got his teeth back. As long as somebody was there with him, things were top-notch. No embarrassment, no apology. Neither of those occurred to

Seamus as a consequence of blindness. For him, helplessness and the occasional fuck-up guaranteed company. In his mind, it was all good. I liked that about him very much.

On our way to his room, prepared to give it all a thorough touch, Seamus knocked a cup over with his cane. He'd left his dentures in water for the night and left the cup on the floor, outside his room. It still seems appropriate. His teeth couldn't wait to get up and talk, just like their owner.

Neither Carson nor Seamus had pretensions. They didn't look at themselves and imagine what the sighted saw or try to be like the sighted. The Aristocrats did both, though. That self-conscious regard causes so much trouble for us, me included. If I walked into a wall in front of someone who sees, I'd be embarrassed. If I did that in front of most people at camp, even though they're blind, too, I'd feel a twinge. More than anything else, I liked Seamus and Carson because I wouldn't feel troubled if they were my audience. They were the kind of blind I hope to be one day. I took that hope with me when I went home early, and we said goodbye.

I didn't have a horrible time at camp, but I'd had enough. I thought my time would have been a lot worse, a lot sweatier, but as I say, I grew to admire a few people, and what they taught me. "Activities" are never something I've sought. Swimming was good, though, and who couldn't enjoy an afternoon of blind people wandering through a stone maze or touching a tree? A really big tree. We didn't gang up on each other's underwear or anything that Cub Scout–nostalgic, but I'd had enough. I will always be the camper who goes home early. That won't change with age or blindness, and it surprised me.

I'd had enough of being blind there, just there, at camp. To live with a group of blind people was tiring. Dedicating our time to activities and conversations that acknowledged, eased, reinforced, or celebrated that we are all of the unseeing kind wasn't enough to keep me in my bunk. Being accommodated was exhausting. I wasn't used to being treated the way a blind person should. I needed a break. Funny enough, going home, to all the sight-centred things of Vancouver, that sounded pretty good. In the city, my blindness is more or less ignored, which helps me ignore it, too.

I came to camp to confront my fear of blind people, and I think I came to some understanding. My cure, I hoped, began with this: there is no such thing as a blind person. That was my discovery, as odd as it may sound. My old horror was that I am, could be, or must become a blind person, as if I could dissolve into that phrase, be that featureless and deleted. But there is no such thing.

Consider the icon for disabled washrooms, the one with the white stick-figure in a wheelchair. It says this room is not for men or women but for the disabled. To know that little wheelchair picture describes everybody and nobody is my new relief. That icon isn't me. It's not Seamus or Cheryl or the Aristocrats or Eddie, either. Stephen Hawking, my former partner, Jane, all the ADHD kids in the world, and Terry Fox are supposed to fit in that same washroom. We're having a big party in here. But few of us have anything more in common than Carson and my brothers or Tracy and Liza might share. As I say, the deaf have a language, which makes community and identity. But other disabilities, like blindness, may fool us into thinking we have our own culture. Disability, in general, likely doesn't have one at all.

Those of us on the island couldn't see. We had that in common. But we couldn't see in such radically different ways, and fashioned such disparate lives out of blindness, that I have to wonder how faked a community can get. Some of us needed the artifice. Seamus did. He needed and enjoyed the island and its support. He'd stay there, if he could. But my need was different. Is different. I needed to go home. I need to always go home in the end. The fear is real. What if, one day, I recognize myself in another blind person? How would I get myself back, then? That was what I use to sweat. How would I get home?

This time, escaping camp was simple enough. I called Tracy. She took the ferry over and picked me up two days early. When I said goodbye to Seamus, he seemed puzzled.

"But camp isn't finished, Ryan. There's two more days."

"I know, but I'm ready to go home. I've got some other things to do."

"But there are two more days," he insisted.

"Tell you what, Seamus. You can have my last two days. They're all yours."

He couldn't believe my naïveté. "You can't give me your two days, silly. I'm already going to be here."

"Well, how about you take my seat in the van, then? The front seat. It's all yours."

The idea pleased him, and he agreed. "Last year I sat in the front seat," he reminded me. "It's a good seat, isn't it?"

"You bet," I said. "Nothing like it."

From what I Hear

I often stop at the Santa Barbara deli on Vancouver's Commercial Drive, a street in the heart of our Little Italy. The deli has a long and busy steel counter, its many glass coolers filled with meats and cheeses of every sort and strength. The place is popular, so you have to take a number and wait your turn, which I do, usually with the help of some other regular who notices me pawing about the countertop for the number tags. Groping raises my notability, and I rely on it as a way of getting help. I'd ask, but sometimes people are as hard for me to locate as the number tags.

Besides the marbled pancetta, what I enjoy most here is the brutal consequence of the deli's speed. When your number comes up, a worker will call it once, twice, and at most three times, and fast. If you happen to be down the aisle some- where squeezing eggplants, well, you're shit out of luck, buddy. Get a new number.

The regulars know that, so we stand alert and on guard. Not even if my number is another three or five away can I afford to feel safe. The regulars like me are easy to spot because we are vigilant, even respectful in our patience, to the coordinated mathematics before us. All day on Sundays we come and go in orderly bunches, stoic and humble, as if waiting for the sacrament itself. It's a terrific dance. Nobody wants to miss their turn.

The Pavlovian imprint is strong and mildly addictive. I get a buzz when my number is called. I've learned to holler "Here! Here!" and wave my tag above the heads around me, heads that smile when somebody else misses a turn. Then, having declared myself "Here!" I move to the counter with a feeling of pride and privilege. I am here, and it is my turn. They are there, and it is not theirs. Somebody else's desires and orders will not be given consideration. Not yet. This is what it means to be called to the counter. It is to be given distinction. Definition from others.

I don't take my deli worker for granted, and I hope she won't take me for granted, either. The next crucial moment to pass between us is when she takes my number and places it on the pile. With this she may say "Hi," or she may say "I'll take that," or "Just a sec," and then she'll step away with my tag. Her work begins, as does mine, now, but my job is specific to blindness.

From those few words I have to form an intimate recognition of her voice. From the four or five others working the counter, I must discern hers alone. When she returns she'll ask, "What would you like?" I may not recognize her voice, and I may, therefore, miss the fact it is me she's speaking to. That happens all the time and makes for a heap of mutual awkwardness. I'll often stare at my deli worker blankly, unaware she spoke to me, while she wonders, perhaps, if I'm lost in an acid flashback, or if I'm deaf.

The blind and sighted difference between us is hard to

explain in the high speed of commercial life. Usually I'll pretend to scratch my nose or rub my temple with the hand in
which I hold my white cane, allowing it to peek above the deli
cases so she'll see I don't see her. But that doesn't guarantee
her use of "Can I help you?" will become any more precise.
As a quick repair, she may see the cane and try to be more
definite with, "What can I get you, sir?" That only slightly
augments my odds of recognizing her voice, what with the
number of sirs with chorizo cravings around here.

What fascinates and spooks me about this crisis is my disappearance. I can vanish into the language others use. Then I
can be found, and I am only found, in specific addresses, not
as "you." I respond to "Can I help you, Ryan?" but not "Can
I help you?"

As a pronoun, "you" assumes I will recognize myself in
language. It assumes I will see the sentence's intention for me
and take it upon myself, for myself, like the beloved, the
intended. But I can't, or I won't.

Too often I have answered questions meant for others
standing beside me. I fail, in this respect, to see myself in the
desires and addresses of others. I don't catch the cues in their
faces, the arrows that give feather and flight to "you" and
direct its meaning at me, and me alone. It is to risk narcissism, then, to take "you" for myself in public spaces and to
thereby admit that I do not know who I am here in relation to
others. "Who are you?" I ask myself. Only "Ryan," in his pre-
cision and familiarity, gives me presence and relation to others. For them, of course, it's an uncommonly overstated need
for distinction.

To refer to another as "you" is to call upon a peculiar arrogance, too. Arrogance means "to claim for one's self." When I am crossing at the corner of Main and Broadway and someone beside me asks, "Hey, where are you going?" I must decide whether to claim the pronoun for myself. If I don't, and the person walking with me waits for my answer, I've suggested that they are not welcome, that their question is invasive and unwanted. That may not be the case at all. On the other hand, if I wait and I hear another voice answer for me, telling me two friends are having a private conversation as they walk, having just bumped into one another at this moment, then I'm correct in leaving the language around me to others.

The arrogance that gives value to the word "you" is always about this predicament. I risk my own misplacement in the world vocalized around me. To not risk it, though, is to disappear myself until I'm given service by my name. It's all very biblical, really. Adam did this for animals, once. God reputedly said, hey, all these critters are going to work for you, just give them all names, first. It makes sense. How else would anybody or anything know when it's their turn?

The other, stranger face of "you" is in my new life as "he" or "him." Even though I require myself to be more distinct in the flow of public movement and more precise in language, some people avoid the problem and bypass me altogether. They may address, as often happens, Tracy instead of me. In that case I'm reduced to the remote social blur of "Would he like a menu?" or "Will you order for him?" It's enough to drive a guy underground.

So I went there. Tracy and I went underground once, one hundred and thirty metres down, on a tour of the salt mines just outside—and, er, under—Krakow. We were on our honeymoon, of course, the kind taken in a Polish salt mine. I wanted to go somewhere dark. That might make it equally memorable for the two of us. Tracy, as always, was game for anything.

First we sat in the mine's main building, patiently waiting for our tour group's turn to descend the original, spiraling wooden staircase into the public chambers. It's a doozy of a walk. The waiting area was solemn and stale smelling, governmental in feel, a lot like the passport office back home. I heard a ticking sound, and Tracy tapped me on the shoulder.

"Hey," she whispered, "it's another blind guy and his wife."

"See?" I said, "I told you this was the place to go. Are they our age?"

"No, older. Fifty, sixty maybe. I don't know. She's sighted, too."

"What if that's us?" I said. "I don't want to meet myself in the future. Not yet."

When the bell rang for everybody to file in for our descent, Tracy steered us into the group near the other blind man. His wife, from her tone, was overjoyed to discover us. Mostly Tracy.

"We should stick together," the woman said. "I'd love the company."

Tracy heard what I heard. By "we" should stick together, this woman referred to herself and Tracy. The blind husband, apparently, couldn't use the company. As for me, I was nowhere to be found.

The four of us neared the entrance to the mine's stairwell.

"Do you want to guide him down first?" the woman asked.

"Who, me?" I said irritably. "I can—" Tracy squeezed my arm, and I shut up. No need to pick an argument here, not now.

So far, not a peep had passed through the blind man's lips. Maybe, in the distant future, I've learned my lesson not to speak unless spoken to. If he was me, I hoped his wife wasn't Tracy. I righted my tone and answered the woman's question for myself.

"No, I'm fine," I answered. "Go ahead and guide your husband. We'll go next."

As Tracy and I entered the stairwell, I felt the claustrophobia I was about to descend into. I also felt the depth of Tracy's. She wasn't exactly keeping it under wraps.

"How many stairs are there, again?" She froze at the first step until I answered.

"Several hundred." More like seven hundred, but I thought "several" was a better expression.

We took the first few steps, and soon the stairwell grew so dark, I couldn't see my usual smudge, not even with the help of the occasional lamp on the wall. It didn't matter to me, though. Stairs are a pattern, and easy. They're a predictable space to move through, unlike nightclubs or South Korea. Tracy put my hand on the railing. I simply followed the wooden line down, easy as pie, one, two, left, right. Easy. Except for the blind guy ahead of us.

Tracy described the scene to me later, so I could better imagine what I'd heard.

As we walked, I could hear the blind man several steps down and ahead of us. His cane struck everything he passed. Hard, too, excessively hard. He wasn't caning, really. More like beating the bush, if there'd been a bush in front of him. According to what Tracy saw, he had no caning style or technique whatsoever. Instead, he used something like a conductor's method, waving the long white stick side to side and up and down, halting in place until he had conducted a clean, four-point sweep of the next step. This slowed everything down to a crawl. Claustrophobia doesn't suffer such impediments well. Nobody could pass him, not without shoving the man aside or down. Everybody had to wait.

It wasn't entirely his doing, either. Tracy said the man's wife was two or three steps below him, walking backwards, holding one of his hands and describing everything as he beat the snot out of it.

"That's right, John, another step, good. Yes, that's the railing, that's the wall, it's clear. And step. Good. Two more and then the landing. Step. Good. That's a lamp." All the while, his cane jerked and spasmed, thwack, thwack, thwack. Even if we'd decided to shove him aside and break for it, the pass wasn't safe. This guy had a weapon. Tracy's claustrophobia was getting worse by the second.

The sound of the cane somehow made the space feel even smaller. It crowded our ears with thwack, thwack, thwack. With little else to do but wait, Tracy made the bona fide mistake of looking down between the staircases. It was lit enough for her eyes to tell her the bottom wasn't anywhere in sight. Her vertigo piled on her claustrophobia, full force, the way I might pile a car on a decorative boulder.

"I think I'm going to freak out," she said. She covered her face with her hands. "I need to go. I need to go now."

Who would've thought someone could get vertigo underground? About ten flights of people clogged the passage behind us. Backing out wasn't an option, not anymore.

"It doesn't sound like we can go back," I said. "Aren't there a lot of people?"

Tracy didn't answer. "Excuse me," she called down to the blind man's wife. "You know, if you let him do it alone, it's easier and we might be able to move a little faster. I'm only saying this out of experience."

Thwack, thwack, thwack.

"It's dark," the man's wife said. "He can't see anything in the dark. Sorry to be so slow, but he needs a guide." She addressed Tracy as a curious and naïve idiot-child, not a vertigo-driven force of nature.

"I don't see in the dark, either," I said, "but it's simple with a hand on the railing to go alone."

Thwack, thwack, clink.

"It's a lamp, John. Step, good."

Tracy pleaded her case. "Maybe you could let John try the railing. I'm not feeling so well." By my calculation, John's wife would not be feeling so well in a moment if Tracy didn't get a move on. "My husband's blind, too, and he actually does better on stairs without a guide."

"That may be," John's wife said, "but I think this works best for him."

Tracy turned to me and whispered in my ear. "What is with this he likes this, he can't do that, I'll help him. I don't do that to you, do I?"

"No, never. It's like the guy isn't there. Hey!" I called to the blind man, "Do you have retinitis pigmentosa?"

The thwacking stopped. "Yes!" John beamed.

"Me too!"

John's pause totally arrested us in the stairwell. I could hear the grumblings from behind. Everybody seemed to imagine the two blind guys were going to hang out and compare war stories.

"You should try hanging on to the railing," I said. "Just hold your cane still at a parallel angle to the stairs. The cane will tap when you're on the bottom step because the tip is lower than you. Stairs are clear—you can trust that."

"Like this," he asked.

"Yes," Tracy answered, then finished the lesson. "Just follow the rail around with your hand when you reach the landings."

Tracy told me the man let go of his wife and began a normal descent, one hand on the railing, the way I was taught. Maybe he'd never had any real mobility instruction, or maybe he'd come very recently to his cane. Then again, if you get too accustomed to someone's guidance, it's hard to let go. Even if it is for a handrail. His wife, in her attempt to be helpful, had taken his hand away from his only functional guide. Not a thwack followed.

When we reached the bottom, we found Mrs. John the Blind Man had, somewhere along the way, decided we shouldn't stick together after all. With her husband's hand on her elbow, she scooted him a few couples away. Some people don't accept guidance well. Or maybe she felt miffed that, by losing her guiding role with John, we'd disappeared her, somewhat.

Our group wandered the dozens of mining chambers, many of which have chandeliers and statuary carved from the rock salt itself. I could taste the salt in the air. At one point, Mrs. John the Blind Man appeared next to Tracy's ear and whispered a sweet reconciliation.

"Is he enjoying the tour?"

"Who?" Tracy said. I was standing beside her.

"Your husband, silly. Is he enjoying the tour?"

"I don't know," Tracy whispered back. "Feel free to ask him."

Mrs. John the Blind Man didn't. Tracy and I were free to resume our honeymoon, and what a spot we were in.

Two brothers, early in the mine's history, had carved an entire underground cathedral from the salt. They excavated tons of the greenish rock and left behind, in its absence, an altar, chandeliers, an ornate and high-vaulted ceiling, statuary, a polished floor, and a descending staircase, all of it salt. I've never heard, smelled, touched, or tasted anything like it.

That's when, once more, I began to dissolve like so much salt. Our tour guide approached Tracy as we walked around the chapel.

"Would he like to touch the statuary?" the guide asked.

Tracy accepted the offer on my behalf. There was no point in arguing with his language. Unlike Mrs. Blind Man, our guide had no reason to know any better about what "he" can do to me.

The feeling is one of deliberate dissociation, becoming "him" all the time. My excavation is performed with the basic tool of a pronoun. In "him," I'm disappeared, instead of brought into definition. "He" is not here, either, like "you." Like me.

The archetype for my problem runs underground, as well. Eurydice struggled with it in Greek mythology. When Orpheus guided her back from the underworld, his most dangerous task was to keep his back to her all the way home, not to look at her or address her until they were both delivered from Hades and up to the light of day above. So much for that prohibition.

When Orpheus, proud of his accomplishment, turned to address his love at the mouth of the cave, Eurydice, still not quite all the way home, was instantly sucked back down and made subterranean. According to Hilda Doolittle's famous poem, Eurydice's reprisal for her disappearance begins with the charge, "For your arrogance." I can dig that. Eurydice was pissed. But who is to answer for it? You? Me? Him?

Not long after we returned from our honeymoon, I noticed myself disappearing in another way. For some time I'd been retreating deeper and deeper into my ears. I'm certain, however, I arrived at a new depth of blindness when a couple of cars crashed outside our apartment. For the first time in my life, I didn't look.

The steely thud happened just below our window, but I
didn't even think to have a gander. Tires squealed, followed
by the smack and crunch of folding metal. Hey, I thought, a
car accident. Then I continued making the bed. I had the
entire story, according to my new body politic. I'd heard
enough to understand all that I could. Unconsciously, I felt
no need to have a look, anymore.

Along with my bigger ears and humbled eyes came a physical and psychological stillness. It stems from the feeling that I
am mired in place, unable to fulfill what sounds ask of me,
which is to look to them. I imagine myself perpetually
stopped in my tracks with one hand cocked to my ear, receiv-
ing signals from the distance. Rarely do I turn my head to the
sounds anymore or go to the window. If I hear a funny noise
in the dishwasher, I tell Tracy about it and wait. I don't
bother to inspect the trouble on my own. The curiosity to go
further isn't in me anymore. And why should it be? My eyes
won't disclose the meaning and cause of the noise, so I just
stay put.

A sound can be an incomplete phenomenon if you don't
have the eyes to go with it. When a noise is made, something
in the world hails us, calls our eyes, and communicates no
other content in its vibrations than that beckoning. But I'm a
short in that circuit. Because I'm not prompted to look, I'm
often left to be still, almost paralysed in listening.

In looking, or looking about, we can be on the go, navigating the oncoming landscape with animated turns of the head,
sometimes pointing and sharing the distance with others,
zooming in and out of places and details with our eyes. We

remain a body in motion, but we are also darting off and away through our eyes, sending out our imaginations into a further space than that taken up with our flesh and bone. Our eyes send us out there, into the distances we look at.

Now I suffer a vital distinction between looking and listening. I live inside the boredom and indifference that comes of a body that only hears. This morning, taking my coffee in a chair by the open living room window, I heard a dog barking somewhere in the neighbourhood. Now and then a car started. The added intrusion of its engine revved and whined, irritating me, until it drove away. The dog continued to bark, however, and I integrated its white noise into my sense of the morning quiet. From where I sat, the sound didn't snag my curiosity or suggest a story of animal abuse I could investigate. It was merely there, in the background.

But, curious about the sound, Tracy walked to our window and looked. Living on the third floor of our building, she could see what was what.

"I saw that dog out there when I went to work yesterday and when I shut the curtains last night. It's so wet. They've left this poor, scrawny lab outside for at least a day and a night now. Assholes."

"Who did?" I asked. "Where?" I imagined the shape of a black lab in various neighbourhood spots.

"That house across the street, the one where all the skaters live."

Tracy stood at the window for a few more minutes, watching the dog. It continued to bark while I finished my coffee and considered who should get first dibs on the tub. My mind was ready to hit the shower, but Tracy's was still out the window, in somebody else's yard.

"Poor dog," she sighed, "it looks so unhappy. It rained last night. It hasn't even got a bowl."

She remained there, perhaps adding up the details of the scene and interpreting the abuse they suggested. No doubt she was right.

My window and Tracy's window are different places, and we are different people with different relationships to the space beyond. Her eyes take her out of the apartment and over to our neighbour's yard. She can watch their dog, place it in the world, and put herself in a story that is happening over there. Seeing encourages that kind of imagination in space. Tracy heard a dog in the distance, which snagged her visual curiosity, and then she looked into it, surveyed the details, inferred a story, maybe even played in it and with the dog in her mind, and then came home, all without leaving the apartment.

But my window only seems to want to let things in, not let me out. I remain a fixed body in space and imagination, unless I force myself to go beyond the sounds in my ears and what I can know that way. In hearing, I receive audible traces from a rough and undetailed world. I hear a dog bark. It is a dog and it is barking, and it is outside somewhere. End of story. I could try to imagine more, but the sound reveals little, making the distance from my window a hefty work of fiction and one slender fact. The dog has no colour, no yard, tidy or unkempt. From what I hear, the dog isn't tethered to a clothesline beside a house with a plastic tarp for a windowpane. Unlike seeing, I can't hear the dog from different angles, to witness its scrawniness. I'm without some curiosity because listening won't do. I have to either be told the details or go across the street to touch everything I can get my hands on and probably get bitten. I can't do any of it from my window. My curiosity is stuck here, inside me.

One afternoon my friend Karina and I were talking over lunch about the aches and pains of student life. You might say we were whimpering about the minor boo-boos that come with reading a lot.

"The nice thing about taped books," I explained, "is that I don't get as much of that scholar's stoop, anymore—you know, from hunching over my desk. Now I just lie in bed and strap on my headset. It's a luxury. The only problem is staying awake."

Karina smiled, I think. "And at least you don't get sore eyes from reading anymore."

"But I do. My eyes are still hardwired into reading. Maybe the ache is from focusing, in its broader sense, but I don't know. About an hour of listening to Martin Amis still gives me a dull pain behind my eyes. I like his fiction, so it isn't the book. It's also not the same kind of ache Canadian novels give me. The British sentences are just, well, just so written. It's like I can't convince my body I'm listening to speech."

That is an old argument Tracy and I have, too. She'll ask me what I'm doing, and I'll say I'm reading. Then she'll say, no you're not, you're listening. Karina had heard that shtick a few times before, so I didn't bother to milk it again.

"I always get muscle aches in my eyes after a few hours of

reading," she said. "Doesn't matter what. The closeness does it. All these words in your face, one at a time and filling your periphery. I love reading, but there's a limit."

Karina would know, too. She's soldiering through her doctoral dissertation, something complex about the history and literary construction of Afro-Canadian settlements in the prairies. To prepare for her two big field exams, she read on average twelve hours a day, every day. I've never regretted bailing on my Ph.D. Occasionally Karina reminds me of at least one reason why—my pain threshold is too low. About as low as my tolerance for academically afflicted writing, the real soul-crushing stuff. I wouldn't want to die with one of those sentences on my mind, and I probably would have.

"There are times," she went on, "when I don't leave my apartment for days. I read for hours without a break and feel like all I want to do is stand in a field and look as far as I can in any direction. I want a view, but I don't want to see anything. I just want something like an eye stretch."

"Why not just shut your eyes?" I asked. "What's the difference?"

"Closing my eyes is too much like nearness, like reading. It's black and it's in your face, sort of crowding you. Gazing down a prairie road stretches me and the muscles in my eyes. I don't necessarily want to see anything. Just look out."

"Like a kind of blindness for the sighted?"

"Exactly," she said and laughed so I would know she was smiling.

In my ears I've known a similar feeling to Karina's crowded eyes. In the restaurant where we'd met, the acoustics were terrible. Large windows and polished concrete floors encouraged noise to ricochet and amplify. On top of that, the owners, like so many hip restauranteurs, drowned the soundscape in deep drum and bass tunes. Rumour is that loud bars and restaurants condition a sense of privacy at a table. Because we can barely hear each other, the implication is that nobody else can eavesdrop.

But, for me, loud noises clutter and impede intimacy, wedging uncomfortably between us. All this bombastic competition for my ears. It pries me from the person with whom I'm speaking. If anything, it manufactures more irksome distance between us. I respond as if someone won't stop waving their hands in my face. Quiet, whatever approximation of silence I can find in the world, is my gaze down a prairie road. Silence is my unfocused view, a space in which my ear stretches to retrieve the furthest irrelevant signal it can detect, just to know how far there is beyond this confined and crowded body of mine. When you are blind, you are always close to your body, imprisoned by its sensory limits.

That's why I often feel stuck, here in my body, here in my office, with an open ear and an open door. I feel as if I've grown stiff, weighted in place, fixed in position, unable to turn my head to a car crash. Because I am out of sight, I imagine myself, to some degree, as out of sight to others. "He" is hidden from view, he is way, way down, somewhere deep within these ears.

Ikealism

Just past Starbucks and McDonald's, Tracy turned our
Honda Civic south. We left Broadway for Knight Street's two
and three lanes of angry eighteen wheelers, all hauling western Canada's supply of galvanized patio furniture, pleather
luggage sets, soda pop syrups, inkjet cartridges and all the
other bumpf of civilization. You name it, you'll find it trucking along Knight Street in Vancouver.

We drove with the windows down and the radio on. The
bold lettering of cube vans promised Tracy's eyes a variety of
expensive personal abstractions. One had all our home reno-
vation needs. Another would motor organic produce to our
door, and a third's red lettering promised a better environment through a cloud of blue exhaust. These monsters sandwiched themselves around our little car and ushered us down
the road. Even though I was in the passenger's seat, it was
loud enough, what with the windows down, that I had to yell
to Tracy, who drove. The fragrant summer air from a few
blocks behind us gave way to a generic stink. I had a question
for my gal.

"Do you think I'm about to come into my own? I'm about
to become a gentleman of property, you know."

I hung my arm out the window, the way my father did when he drove with one hand. I remember how he relaxed in this pose with a cigarette. He's quit smoking recently, and although my eyes keep me from driving, only a shred of will keeps me from smoking. I hung my arm out the window anyway, trying to resemble the image I have of adulthood in a car.

"Well, how do I look? Don't I look like a man about to be a man of means?"

Tracy didn't examine me. She looked in the rearview mirror and brushed her bangs. I think she did.

"'Gentleman of property'? Gentleman in itself is a stretch, but you're about to buy a sofa, bub. I don't think owning a sofa makes you a gentleman of property."

I drew my arm back into the car and reached for the tuner button on the radio.

"Couch," I corrected, "we're going to buy a couch, not a sofa."

The stereo's blurry face plate glowered at me from the dashboard. It made me think of the storm trooper helmets from *Star Wars*. I pressed its right eye and waited for the tuner to scan and find a song appropriate to our quest for a new couch, our initiation into big ticket ownership.

The tuner stopped on the local university station. A band of three or four men mumbled through an interview about their group's particular sound. One of them described a blend of calypso, punk, and techno-bluegrass. "Yes, yes," the interviewer agreed, all espresso and enthusiasm. "I can hear that," he said. I couldn't.

"Why not a sofa?" Tracy asked and changed the station. "Sofas and couches are the same thing."

Joni Mitchell's voice piped through the speakers. In her high, breezy flutter she sang that chorus about paradise and parking lots. When I was a kid and I heard this song on the radio in my mother's station wagon, I always thought Mitchell was saying "they paid paradise to put up a parking lot." I'd wondered who Paradise was and why he made parking lots. The song never resonated with me much. I screwed up my face at Tracy's question and Mitchell's falsetto.

"We're not buying a sofa," I said. "Sofas are American. Jesus, I hate this song."

"And couches are Canadian? What about chesterfields?"

"British. We're probably closer to chesterfields than sofas, but I don't think IKEA would have anything I'd call a chesterfield. Sounds too majestic. Swedish minimalism is never that decadent."

I reached out and changed the station again, jumping through four call-in shows before switching to FM.

"A couch," I added, "is what we're buying. That's a term for chesterfield with common sense."

Continuing south, we were about to cross the Knight Street Bridge. I still hadn't found the right soundtrack. I thumbed the scan button again, this time landing on a local locker room guitar station. If you listen long enough, it's clear these stations only rotate four or five emo-metal songs per day, but we were running out of choices, so I stopped scanning for a loathsome moment.

Emo-metal, or "emotional metal," is the marketing term for this generation's own saccharine, power-chord enemas. It's clearly art for commerce students, but we had to listen because I sometimes like to quiz Tracy's pop culture repertoire. One of those typical angst bands, the kind with a single-word name, belted out some sludge about how they were all fixing to die because nobody understood them. Or something in that ballpark. I couldn't understand the words. The quiz began.

"Now, listen here, buddy, which of the many emo-metal bands are we currently enjoying? In the spirit of modern education, I'll give you a multiple choice format. Is this composition by (A) Creed, (B) Staind, (C) Moist, or, tricky, tricky, (D) none of the above?"

Tracy gave pause and tipped her head back, as if taking in an unidentified smell. If I know Tracy's face, I bet it puckered, as if noting crap in the air.

"I don't know. Uh, is it Moist?" She squeezed the word out in two syllables like a blob of toothpaste. "Moy-yist. What a horrible word."

"Final answer?"

She didn't say anything, then added, "Yup, sorry." She'd probably nodded.

"Oh, I'm so, so sorry, Moist is not the answer. Moist is not even an emo-metal band."

She hit me on the shoulder, "Yes they are!" Thump. I felt like a TV with bad reception. "Moist is too an emo-metal band." Double thump.

"No, the literature says Moist is an art-rock band with some pretense to gothic roots. Mostly because of their cryptic and stupid lyrics about how macabre human nature is. This is Staind, buddy, Stay-nd, Christian rock, admittedly, but emo-metal made flesh. Tune your delicate ear to the differences here. You can tell emo-metal from something like Moist because, without the music, emo-metal vocals sound like New Country. It drives the emo-metalheads nuts when you point this out. Garth Brooks could do this stuff, if he wanted, and he pretty much does."

Tracy punched another button on the storm trooper's face. A classic rock station came in, the one that has two male deejays who tell fart jokes and coyly allude to liking dope. George Thorogood played his version of John Lee Hooker's "One Bourbon, One Scotch, and One Beer." The station's ball-scratching hosts burst into song, making it their own. "One Cuban, one Scotch, and one quee-eer . . ."

We both punched the radio's off button.

By now we were on the Knight Street Bridge, crossing the Fraser River from Vancouver to the suburb of Richmond. Tracy checked the side view mirror and turned the car into the outer lane, ready to exit when we reached the other side. At mid-span I looked out my window and down at the flat brownish waters. The blinding fluid in my retinas mingled and matched with the river's motion, or what I imagined must be there, the waves of light and shape in my eyes wiping the river's lively detail into a flat brown sheet. A brown paper bag of water. I scanned to the edges of the empty bag and up into a large cluster of featureless wavy blocks. Warehouses, I thought, not tall enough for office buildings. Maybe a few malls. From a distance it was hard to determine the difference. That goes for a lot of things.

"Oh, I wish you could see this," Tracy jeered. "I knew it. There's the sign." She pointed at the blocks. "You thought I couldn't find it, but it's right there, chump, in yellow and blue, so you can stop knotting-up inside about getting lost."

I have to admit Tracy does have an uncanny clairvoyant power for finding places. I've never seen her open a map, and I've tried to thrust a few into her hands. Once I bought a map as a less-than-covert gift from a gas station somewhere near Sooke, on Vancouver Island.

"Here's your Happy Planet juice, some chips and—look!—I got us a map."

She feigned thankfulness and binned her new map in the glove box. We pulled out of the gas station as she assured me that the resort is just over here somewhere. When Tracy says whatever we're looking for is just over here somewhere, it means we'll drive half an hour in some general direction and, eerily, pull into the best parking spot, not a wrong turn from start to finish. Indeed, I gave up driving when I started driving into things, but I never gave up trying to control the wheel.

The morning Tracy asked me if we ought to go to IKEA to buy a couch, I should have known better than to ask if she knew where the closest IKEA was located, exactly.

"It's in Richmond. Somewhere in Richmond."

She stood in our cramped little bathroom, a bag of cosmetics in hand. Putting on her makeup while asking if we should buy a couch meant she'd already made up her mind that we were going to IKEA today, and asking me if we ought to go was her way of saying "Get your shoes on." It's dizzying, all the versions of meanings available to the listener.

I hung around in the bathroom doorway for a minute and watched her draw a thin, defining line of colour around her lips. In my eyes the line she drew, the ends of her lips, eyes, chin, nose, and hair, all the defining edges of her face, rippled wildly as if someone had just tossed a stone in the reflecting pool of her image.

"IKEA is somewhere in Richmond?" I scoffed. "We're going to jump in the car and drive to somewhere in Richmond to buy a couch?"

She snapped her makeup case shut. "Precisely."

Now she'd found the store, spying it from the bridge, and within minutes here we were, parked three spots from the door, right next to the handicapped spaces. I don't know how she does it.

Pause for a moment just inside an IKEA entrance and close your eyes. You'll notice the air at any IKEA has that same ubiquitous blend. A lot of information and marketing is communicated through that smell, but the demands placed on our vision by the cornucopia of furniture and gizmos is usually too much to let anybody really put a nose to work. What's most striking is the uniformity of that smell, no matter which location you find yourself in or where you are in the vast warehouse space. The odour is always the same cheap cocktail of vinyl, pine, plastic, particleboard, and cotton, always distinct but never unique.

Tracy and I entered through the store's automatic doors. The air immediately clung to us, travelled with us, and made a veritable biosphere of manufactured smell. What the uniformity in my nose says is this: hey, relax, there are no wrong turns in IKEA. Everything goes here. Nothing is bold or discrete enough to be out of place, mismatched, or in need of judgment. All your needs can be found in this jigsaw of compatible smells, all of it under warm track lighting. No design is necessary, and there is no need to imagine a future or variation. IKEA is a total and enclosed system of comfort. Smell it, dig it, relax in it.

Beyond the automatic doors we spelunked into a connected cavern of sound. I could hear strollers, arguments, bin clatter, heels on laminate flooring, each sound nearby and distant, all at once. No matter how closely you attend to individual sounds, here and there are irrelevant ideas, both indistinguishable to the ear in IKEA.

Space gives away, too. The blind measure space by time travelled through it, instead of by sights as they pass. That's why IKEA and malls in general are havoc for me. In IKEA Tracy and I move forward and sideways, pause and push on. Then we retrace steps to go back and compare prices and colours. The wandering design gives me the illusion that, at each bend in the path, space replicates itself. It is not one room but many rooms and many more rooms, each without an indication of what could come next. No sign of exit or entry can be detected, so the focus is singular. Shop. Or in my case, get lost.

I took Tracy's elbow, and we weaved past the ballroom and up the stairs and started our search for the couch zone. The odor and noise and darting crowds were already too much for me. By the time we reached the home office furnishings, I'd already become somewhat of a crank. Actually, belligerent.

"So this is where the neighbourhood went," I sneered. "They put a roof over it, took the walls off the stores, and made it one big safari walk."

"I guess so," Tracy said. She sounded preoccupied. She was looking for things.

"Why do you think they want everybody to dehydrate in here? Maybe the real money in IKEA is made at the ice cream stand at the end. It's so goddamn dry."

I took a few more snide potshots, even described my boredom, until Tracy had heard enough and told me so.

"Look, if you're going to tag along just to throw barbs, I'll take my elbow back and let you do this on your own. It may not be fun for you, but we need to buy a sofa."

"I'm just joking around."

"Sure, but you always do this. We need a sofa but—"

"Couch," I said.

"Whatever. We need one, but as soon as we walk into a store, you immediately begin to snarl at everything. It's not fun for me, you know."

"Well, it's not fun for me either," I said. "I don't see anything in here. My day is gonna be me being dragged around for a couple of hours, as if I have any opinion on this stuff. It all looks the same to me. Wavy."

Tracy was frustrated and jerked her elbow out of my hand.

"Why can't you at least indulge me a little?" she asked. "I like doing this. I like to shop, sometimes. If it all has to be about you, stay home and let me enjoy this if I want to. I like to find things for our home. Is that so bad?"

I didn't want to argue, especially not with us clogging the aisle the way we were.

"Fine." I said. "I'll keep my boredom to myself. Sorry for not getting into the whole IKEA thing."

But I wasn't sorry, that much we both understood. We could at least move on to the couches and, hopefully, home.

Tracy gave me her elbow again, picked up her pace, an aggressive driver, and towed me around couples as they exited into the pit stops of complete bedroom displays. I squinted at the displays, a blandness of distortion, and felt, for some reason, my annoyance begin to dissipate. We skipped from display to display, just as we'd jumped from radio station to radio station. The front lines of my resistance receded with every picture frame and knickknack I picked up. I was acclimatizing.

Like most people, I suspect, I've often wondered if I could live in IKEA. Certainly everything I need is here. Once again I picked up the thread of that idea and followed it around my mind. Doing it was at least an amusing way to substitute for the lack of variation in smell and sound.

Maybe I could pitch my services as a living model. I could be employed to live here and show interested customers what it looks like to pass your time in various displays.

"See the peaceful expression on our model's face as he sleeps on a blond, pine, queen-sized bed complete with head-board and autumn print duvet and pillow cases? How much do you think he paid for that peaceful expression? $800?"

From under blankets, I'd stir and yawn on cue, breaking the theatrical fourth wall.

"Good morning! I sleep well at night knowing I paid only $499 for this complete set."

My job, as a living model, would both advertise a dull and affordable IKEA lifestyle and model disabled independence for interested government and nonprofit agencies. IKEA could employ disabled people around the world to live in their stores. IKEA would be a sort of school for disabled youth. Students would come to study strategies for independent living, then take up a short residency as a practicum. Module One: Kitchen Life, Module Two: Bedroom Ergonomics, and so on. IKEA would receive, in turn, a warmhearted and socially supportive PR image.

I was busy mulling over this idea when Tracy abruptly exited the store's thoroughfare and eased us into an oasis of chairs, stools, and couches. She signaled me to let go with a slight lift of her arm. I dropped her elbow. Quickly she maneuvered around the couches, narrowing the field of choices. Waiting, I opened my white cane and floated about the aisles, a free radical obstructing the flow of customers through the IKEA bloodstream.

Tracy called me over, and I followed her voice to a large brown glob between a number of other large brown globs.

"What do you think of this one?"

I stared at the brown shape for what I estimated to be a thoughtful moment. Pretending to inspect the goods, I walked around the couch. I scratched my chin and hmmmed under my breath. If the brown glob had tires, I would have kicked them.

"I don't know," I said, as if juggling a myriad of decisive factors. I put my hand on the upholstery. The cushions felt puffy and more or less couch-like. I sat on it. No sound, a slight give in the cushions, nothing surprising.

"Well," I said decisively, "you can comfortably sit upright, and it's relatively long, so I'm going to say it must be a couch."

"Duh, but what do you think of the colour?"

Tracy knows I can see some colour, but sometimes it's unclear, when she asks for my opinion, if it is done more out of duty to that bit of sight I have left or out of a sincere belief in my judgment. In the past I have worn purple and green, claiming they were blue and gray. The colour of this couch was fairly black and white, though.

"Brown?" I asked. "What is there to think about brown?"

"I really like the colour, " she said.

"Brown? What's so great about brown?"

"No, buddy, this isn't brown, this is camel."

I screwed up my face the same way I do at emo-metal.

"Camel? I hate beige."

Tracy hauled me off the couch and over to another. "This," she said, "this is more of a beige, and that's camel. There's a big difference."

I looked at the two brown things.

"Oh, I see. Well, what about that one?" I asked, pointing to another couch. "Or is that the same one I was just sitting on?"

"That's more of an oatmeal colour. Or maybe sand."

"Sand? Is that off-white?" I tried to remember my favourite t-shirt from grade nine, a large, ill-fitting man's undershirt my mother told me was off-white when I'd always seen it as a plain white shirt. It still looked white in my mind. White always did.

"Sort of off-white," Tracy answered, "but more like a cream colour, almost, but less yellow. Oh, hey! Let's look at those ones over there."

I sat down on a brown couch and looked at all the other brown couches. "You let me know when you've narrowed it down. I don't think I'm much use here." She left me to my thoughts, which were in many ways more comfortable than the couches. My thoughts each had a texture, shape, colour, and intensity, or lack of intensity, I could discern and savour. The couches didn't.

Physically, blindness leaves me here in a world where I am only certain about shapes and textures. All I could see were couches, but little else to distinguish one from the other. I still hated shopping and hated how generic the world appeared to my senses.

An old man in a blue IKEA shirt flopped heavily down on the cushion next to me. Maybe it was a green shirt. I don't know. He stretched and relaxed, legs splayed in front of him, obviously someone on a break. On his chest was a magnetic name tag. I pieced the letters together in the clean sliver of my good eye. I read just as I did in grade two. One letter at a time, then sounded them out together.

"Excuse me," I said, "does your name tag say Plato?"

He folded his arms and grunted in affirmation.

"*The* Plato? As in *The Republic*?"

"You've read it?" he asked, a hint of surprise in his voice. "Boy, that dates a man."

"And you work here?" I asked.

"Sure do. You need help?"

I wasn't clear what kind of help he was offering. A better defence for having kicked poets out of his republic would be a good start, but a hand with the couch choices might be more appropriate to the moment.

"Can I ask you something?" I said.

He put his hands behind his silvery head and crossed his long, bony fingers.

Who am I kidding? I have no idea what he did. I just heard him move in his seat.

"Sure, as long as it's not a counselling question. I'm not a counselor. I saw you and your wife or girlfriend debating here. I don't handle that."

"Huh?"

"You know, the counsellors, that's their turf. It's off-season. Don't you know about them?" I shook my head. "During the pre-Christmas rush, management hires a gang of marriage counsellors to roam the store and help customers who might be feeling stressed about large purchase decisions. Management asked me to supervise the service. They thought my so-called skills inventory made me the perfect candidate to supervise a team of self-help lemonade stands. Makes me sick. I'd rather stock can openers. This is between you, me, and these brown couches, though, okay? Anyways, how can I help you?"

Obviously he was on his break, so I opted not to ask about the couches. But since I had Plato's ear, which is better than sitting next to Freud on the couch, I wanted to keep him talking.

"I wanted to ask, well, I just wanted to know how you like working here."

"It's okay. The benefits package could use some work, but the people are nice. The whole experience has me thinking some ideas over again."

Tracy called from farther down the aisle. She wanted to know if we were going to buy a matching chair or not. I said I'd be there in a second. Plato had taken a notepad and pen from his shirt pocket. I could hear the pen scratching as he made notes.

"What could IKEA possibly make you reconsider?"

"Well," he began and flipped a few pages back through his notepad. He read a little, looked up, and pulled on his beard with a fidgety tug. "Well, something went wrong. I'm concerned that this is the kind of place where the Republic ought to have begun, at least in a small way. I'd like to think we are selling some of the day-to-day infrastructure for a utopia here, but I'm not so sure anymore."

I squinted and surveyed the room, trying to see utopia. "I'm sorry, but I don't see it," I said.

Plato pointed to my white cane. "Do you have any sight?" he asked.

"Just shapes and a bit of light and colour. Not much more than wavy shadows, really."

"I bet you see what I mean," he said. "Think of it this way. There should be no competition here. You can't go wrong. It's basically all the same. I wish people would see that."

I looked at the sea of brown couches again. "So, you guys sell me one version of everything here, with only minor variations? Is that what you mean?"

"More or less," he agreed. "It gives folks some harmless sense of choice and individuality. We sell what I call Ikealism. Not a chair or a lamp, but chairness and lampness."

"Like Cabbage Patch Kids."

Plato wasn't up on his 1980s pop culture.

"They were dolls," I explained, "cute and creepy dolls with detailed heads. You could kind of see a fundamentally universal Cabbage Patch face, but each one was marketed as having at least one minor computer-generated difference. That made each one singular and worthy of its own name. Also made them cost a mint. I think some parents died fighting over them."

"They came with names?" Plato asked.

"Birth certificates, too. My little sister had one named Roger Igor. For a while, anyway. My brothers cooked him one day on the barbecue. My sister found out when she saw the video."

Plato muttered something, and I heard his pen scratching.

"You realize," he said as he wrote, "that you are scripting a conversation in which you not only put words into Plato's mouth, but you have offered him a Cabbage Patch Kid analogy?"

"What's your point?"

From the chair across from us he took two pillows and held them up. One was red and the other blue. I think. The shape and texture were the same, although one was bigger than the other.

"I had said once," he explained, "that the artisans, along with the artists, had to leave the Republic because they're all liars. They make, with their crafts and their poems and sculptures, artful variations on the shadows of ideal forms. Imitations are lies, and lies ain't good."

"Even a table is a lie?" I asked.

"It's a version of the ideal table, so it's a lie."

In my mind I pictured a utopia in which everybody sat on rocks and ate with their hands. My time at scout camp came back in all its utopian horror.

"The individuality of things," Plato continued, "their distinction, is what we see people coveting today. That's one of the many sources of inequality. Unchecked individualism. The pursuit of "me" and "mineness." But I think for people to be equal, first, all things—our material conditions—must be equal. IKEA expresses an unsophisticated idea of that promise. Yet, somehow we failed to make an equality of things here, even though little or no uniqueness is available to fight over."

I agreed. I couldn't see anything but brown couches. Why anybody would choose one over another was beyond me.

"I don't mean to bore you with all this," Plato said, "but my conclusion is short. The irony is we can't manufacture away individualism. It is seen even when it isn't there. So I was wrong. What can I say? I eat my crow when it's served. Artisans and their trades don't make versions or make lies, after all. It was never in the objects themselves but in the seeing, in people's desires to see something unique, no matter what."

Tracy called again, and Plato got up with me. He excused himself to finish his break in peace, maybe just on another couch. I thanked him for the chat and listened to him wander away.

What came over me next, definite and bright, was a deep and urgent sense of my affection for Tracy. I wanted to apologize, find her among the maze of couches, and help her choose one. I had been a jerk of sorts, a smug blind guy in IKEA, as if I were outside it all. Cynicism wasn't the right exit, nor was righteousness. With Tracy I can feel a necessary relief from my individuality, from blindness, from all my differences, be they subtle or bold. That's a better way out of here.

I knew, and I continue to know, her pleasure should be mine, be it sand, beige, or brown, wherever I can find it, whatever shape and colour it may take for her. It doesn't matter if it is a couch or a poem or a city. To not want to see what she is looking for, even if I can't, that is my worst crime against my Republic. I have to want to see what's out there for her, with her, although it's not there for me or my eyes. That's only fair to our differences.

When I found her near a brown glob of couchness, I asked

her to describe it to me. As it came into focus, with each word, IKEA disappeared around us, its couches and its smell, and left me alone with Tracy's voice. I coveted every word of her.

Losing Face

Vladimir: "When did this happen to you?"
Pozzo: "I don't know. . . . The blind know nothing of time."
    —Samuel Beckett, *Waiting for Godot*

I haven't seen my face in five years.

Because I haven't seen it, I've awakened into a new order, a different sense of time and identity, like a strange twist on those bad made-for-TV flicks. You know the ones. Some poor schmuck is struck by an ambulance, lands in a coma, and wakes up a dozen years later to face a stranger in the mirror. Blindness is a kind of inverted coma. I wake up everyday with Peter Pan in my smile. I look in the mirror, but the person looking back remains young and not there, just an idea. The world gets older, but I see no evidence of it. I see no evidence of time writing itself on my face, either.

It seems strange to live a life but never reveal your final face. Most of us are afraid of it. We're haunted by the idea that one morning we will discover an old person in the mirror. But I'm afraid of how I will make peace with that absence. I never saw my time coming and never will.

I haven't seen the faces of others in years, either. Some people, those new to me at the college where I teach or around the coffee shop where I don't teach, they're without faces, except the caricatures and portraits my imagination doodles. Others from my sighted past, such as my parents, my brothers and sister, and Tracy, their faces remain lit in my mind but also eerily suspended in time, along with my own.

What I did not expect, nor could I have anticipated, was the loss of my face to others. Because I don't see faces anymore, mine included, I seem to have, well, stopped giving face. I'm giving up on its expressiveness, its animated reactions to the world, despite knowing others look at my expression and can spot it quite well. You could say I'm losing touch with my face, even losing some control of it. If you don't receive the facial expressions of others, you forget to give back in kind.

Tracy will ask me what's wrong when I'm quiet and content, maybe listening to the radio or entertaining an idea. Inside I'm engaged by what I'm hearing around me, experiencing pleasure in the textures of thought or the surrounding fracas of restaurant talk, but I look pissed off. My face characterizes me as serious and dour, even consistently angry, according to my students. But that isn't how I feel. I've simply forgotten my face. I'm not indifferent or retreating from the world around me but from my face itself.

Somewhere in my family's tooled wooden chest of memorabilia, kept behind a plastic slip in a cloth-bound photo album, is a picture of me. A young me. A seeing me. It was taken by my father when I was ten years old.

If I lift this photograph up and hold it close to the shrinking island of vision in the centre of my right eye, I can see, scanning the picture, bits of lawn, a shoeless foot—toes, mostly—high in the left corner, something red, a knee towards the centre, a ball, and above that, about an inch higher in the photo, perhaps a quarter of my young face, the left eye and nose and a bit of my forehead. Each of the fragments I see is smaller than a dime. If I look at the word "dime" on this page, less than half of the letter "m" is clear to me. My tunnel vision is that narrow now. Total blindness is that near.

Dragging the rake of my eye around that backyard photo, I collect holes of clarity. They are coins of shape and resemblance similar to the paper bites taken by a three-hole punch. With a little time and patience, I can piece them together in my mind and infer what used to be a cohesive scene from my life.

The picture holds a moment in time I remember and remember seeing. Playful, ten-year-old shenanigans we had in the backyard. I have a memory, and I have a photo of it. I am, however, becoming blind to both. My eyes and my mind's eye are deteriorating. Together.

What you might see is a picture of a potbellied kid in red shorts, shirtless and shoeless, grinning, winding up for a pitch with a muddy softball in his right hand. The angle of the camera suggests the photo was taken from above. The top of a wooden railing in the bottom of the picture suggests it was taken from some kind of veranda. My brother Rory, five years old, barefoot in green shorts and a white t-shirt, is running away from the camera or from me as I threaten to let the ball go. My pitch would head straight for the lens, if my aim was any good, and if I'd actually thrown the ball that day.

Although I don't see all this in the photograph at once, I remember the details. How I remember them, though, is changing. Contracting.

Description is a lot of work. You at least get a sense of the patience required to reconstitute a sight from its pieces—and I've only sketched out the most general of resemblances here. I've said nothing about textures, expressions, shadow, landscape, and so on. All that could be communicated instantly if I'd just printed the picture for you. But that would miss the first point.

My eyes, with only 1 percent of a functioning retina left, arrange visual experience in a manner more like narration than "seeing." My world is gathered up like so many fragmented descriptions that, hopefully, accumulate one at a time into something clear and whole and real. Like a book. When you read my description of a picture, you come to see it as I do: in pieces.

If you'll indulge me just a smidge longer, I agree that there is little evidence so far of a profoundly meaningful photograph, one that is weighty enough to conclude my memoir, my autopathography. The backyard picture wasn't figurative in the beginning of my blindness. It doesn't connect to the day I was diagnosed or the image I saw when I discovered the eroding holes in my visual field. Yet this picture always stuck in my mind's eye and conjures an acute memory in my body of that mischievous surge I felt when I wasn't sure if I would let the ball go at my father's camera. That would have been just like me, pushing the joke too far. That memory in my body is still a clear picture, although the picture in my hand is not.

The moment is as good as any to show how blindness is a verb, a blinding, which may be only that. My blindness is without a defined ending. I am a blinding man. Unfinished. Maybe perpetual.

At the time of my backyard goofing, in 1983, I could see a lot. I had healthy eyes, and to this day they leave a phantom sensation of what it was like to live inside a seeing body. I saw my father's moustache poking out from under the camera, his tree-like forearms and chest. I recall the ease of my eyes gathering in the periphery, taking in the weight of my father's body as he leaned back a bit on his left foot in his brown sandals and summer denim cutoffs. The deck below him was painted brown, as was our house's wooden siding, white shutters framing each window, a barbecue under tarp beneath one of the windows. The light and colour flanked further down. Without moving my eyes, I could take in the edge of the lawn below the deck, and the oily, brown railroad ties that divided the thick green lawn from the concrete patio. Above it all my father stood and asked us to say cheese. One piece at a time, I try to rebuild the memory of what I once saw in a single flash of light.

Now, when I look at any picture from my past, a frightening exchange of time happens. What I saw in my life with good eyes, I can no longer remember without blinding it, cutting memories up into the confetti of my present condition. As the disease eats away at my retina, as it eats into the future, it is also eating its way back through my mind's eye and all it saw, full and well, in the past. When I was ten, I saw my father with his camera. Now I remember him that day as if, back then, I was this man who is on the edge of total blindness.

I dream in tunnel vision, I think. I remember in tunnel vision, I think. The question remains, when my tunnel vision goes, as it will very soon, what will I remember seeing? How will I remember?

All I can do is write it down and keep writing. How else can I hold this picture, this life, or this face together? The view from here is of a boy with a softball, ready to let it go. His is an ironic gift from the past, as if the young me is aiming at the old, saying, "Here, buddy, let me help you with that." I wanted to let the ball fly at my lens, whatever was left of it.

My hope is that one day soon I'll puzzle over another ten-year-old boy. Or maybe it will be a girl. Tracy and I would be thrilled either way. Because I'm thinking about my father taking a picture of his son, let's just say, for fun, that it's a boy. I've got an image in mind, I think.

When the time is right, I'll show him this photograph of me and my softball and let him find some of his young face in my own. In our family, only Tracy will play baseball with our son, and only Tracy will take the family photos. To him I will tell all the stories, of things I've seen and things I've never seen.

Then, one day, my son will ask me the inevitable question, "How long have you been blind?"

I'll try to recall what I've seen in my life and try to remember exactly when the images stopped visiting me. I worry that I already know the answer, though.

"I've been blind," I'll have to say, "for as long as I can remember."

Acknowledgements

I am grateful to the following friends, family, readers, editors, writers, and strangers for helping me realize this book, and its blindness, as my own:

Lane Bergeson and the *Utne Reader;* George Bowering; Mark Cochrane; Wayde Compton; Brad Cran; Michael Davidson; Jennifer, Perry, and Jack Gray; Joanne Hoedemaker; John Hull; Bobby Ixnay; Gillian Jerome; Reg Johanson; Georgina Kleege; Erin Knighton, the Coma Girl; Mykol Knighton, who fixed my pants; Rory Knighton, missed; my parents, Miles and Kathie, who never, ever flinch; the tooth and cure of Jim Knipfel; Jason Le Heup; Ashok Mathur, for the test run at the Emily Carr Institute of Art and Design; Don McKellar, who read the first and unforgivably long draft; Stan Persky, for our metaphysical car pool; Paul Pigat, for the riffs between; Helen and Tony Rawa; Eden Robbins; Gary Ross and *Saturday Night Magazine;* the sentences of Oliver Sacks; the revelatory horror of Jose Saramago; Slickity Jim's Chat and Chew, for the soup and space; Scott Smith; George Stanley; Anne Stone; Sharon Thesen and the *Capilano Review;* Will Trump, my first teacher in blindness; Michael Turner; Peter Van Garderen; Karina Vernon; Alana Wilcox and the folks at Coach House

Books; my colleagues at Capilano College, who, for some reason, hired me when my fly was down; the generous and forgiving people at blind camp; and that guy at the pub who told me I needed to take responsibility for bumping into him. Consider it done.

I owe a unique debt, a large tab, to Brian Fawcett at Dooneyscafe.com, whose encouragement and curiosity coaxed this book, sentence by sentence, and who first edited me into an understanding of my blindness.

For her spirited advocacy of my writing, not just my story, I am extremely grateful to my agent, Denise Bukowski, and all the folks at The Bukowski Agency.

To my editors, Lisa Kaufman at PublicAffairs and Diane Turbide at Penguin, my awe and thanks for finding rabbits in my hat. My gratitude extends to all the people at both presses for putting their shoulders to this thing.

Much gratitude remains, and I give it all to Tracy Rawa, for her love, patience, friendship, strength, humour, and unrivalled bullshit detection.

PublicAffairs is a publishing house founded in 1997. It is a tribute to the standards, values, and flair of three persons who have served as mentors to countless reporters, writers, editors, and book people of all kinds, including me.

I. F. Stone, proprietor of *I. F. Stone's Weekly,* combined a commitment to the First Amendment with entrepreneurial zeal and reporting skill and became one of the great independent journalists in American history. At the age of eighty, Izzy published *The Trial of Socrates,* which was a national bestseller. He wrote the book after he taught himself ancient Greek.

Benjamin C. Bradlee was for nearly thirty years the charismatic editorial leader of *The Washington Post.* It was Ben who gave the *Post* the range and courage to pursue such historic issues as Watergate. He supported his reporters with a tenacity that made them fearless, and it is no accident that so many became authors of influential, best-selling books.

Robert L. Bernstein, the chief executive of Random House for more than a quarter century, guided one of the nation's premier publishing houses. Bob was personally responsible for many books of political dissent and argument that challenged tyranny around the globe. He is also the founder and was the longtime chair of Human Rights Watch, one of the most respected human rights organizations in the world.

.   .   .

For fifty years, the banner of Public Affairs Press was carried by its owner Morris B. Schnapper, who published Gandhi, Nasser, Toynbee, Truman, and about 1,500 other authors. In 1983 Schnapper was described by *The Washington Post* as "a redoubtable gadfly." His legacy will endure in the books to come.

Peter Osnos, *Founder and Editor-at-Large*